Medicine in Brief
Volume 2

Medicine in Brief
Volume 2

NAME THE DISEASE IN
HAIKU, TANKA AND ART

CYNTHIA COOPER, MD
Illustrations by Pamela Chen, MD

Haiku and Tanka are traditional forms of Japanese poetry. Haiku are structured as three lines with 5-7-5 syllables. Tanka have five lines with 5-7-5-7-7 syllables.

The poems are stereotypes of diagnoses and do not reflect the full spectrum of disease or patient experience. The explanations contain medical information but should not substitute for advice from a physician.

Dedicated to my husband who always knew I could.

Puzzles to be solved
Exam, labs, pictures involved
History's the key

Best teacher haiku
Prune back old, extend the new
Bonsai Medicine

Foreword
Maegaki

This book is designed to celebrate the language of medical history and diagnosis. The reader is asked to consider the poem on the right-hand page as a riddle. What is the possible diagnosis? How do the words lead toward a certain pathophysiology? Turn the page. On the following left-hand page is a brief explanation of the clues and the subject of the poem. Readers are encouraged to use this book as a springboard from which to continue their own study.

Forward
Zempo

CONTENTS

Cardiopulmonary	11
Infectious Disease	63
Rheumatology	115
Endocrinology	143
Gastroenterology/Hepatology	169
Nephrology	193
Integumentary	213
Gynecology/Genitourinary	263
Hematology/Oncology	279
Neurology/Psychiatry	309
Acknowledgements	353
Index	355

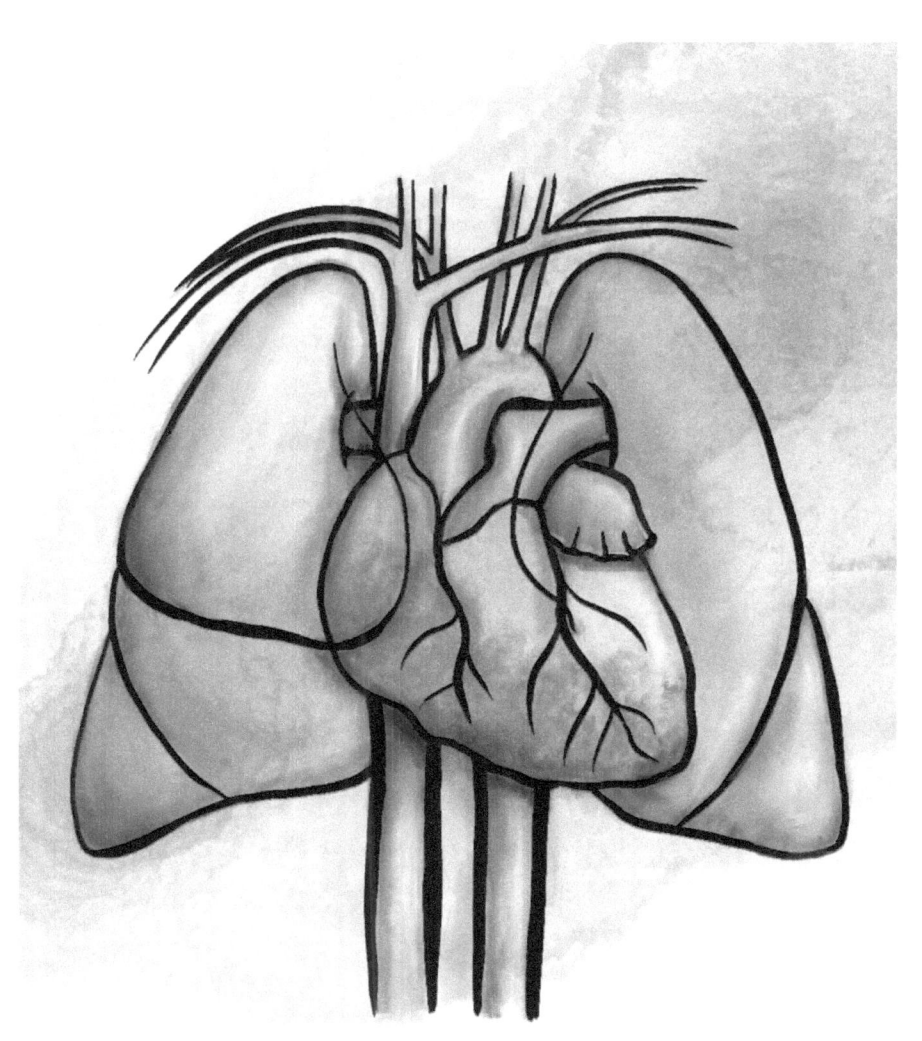

Cardiopulmonary

Cardiopulmonary
Shinhai

By breath and by beat
Fuel for raging fire complete
Two entwined circles

Undulating trace
Twirling, turning points in space
Last beat long QT
Hypo K or hypo Mag
Risk from what makes repol lag

Torsades de Pointes

Torsades de pointes (TdP) is French for 'twisting of the points.' This polymorphic ventricular tachycardia has a sine wave superstructure to the tracing on an electrocardiogram (ECG). TdP is associated with either a congenital or acquired long QT interval, such as from low potassium, low magnesium, drugs, ischemia, or bradycardia. Unstable TdP, e.g., with hypotension or hypoperfusion, is managed with advanced cardiac life support (ACLS). Stable TdP is treated with boluses of IV magnesium, correction of electrolyte abnormalities and discontinuation of any provoking medications.

Fibrofatty change
With each year, scar spreads its range
Warped V1 through 3
VT sparked by exercise
'Walk don't run,' words to the wise

Arrhythmogenic Cardiomyopathy

Arrhythmogenic cardiomyopathy (ARC), previously known as Arrhythmogenic Right Ventricular Dysplasia, is a familial, mostly autosomal dominant cardiomyopathy. The myocardium is slowly replaced with fibrofatty scar, starting in the right ventricle, but often spreading to the left heart. Expansion of the scar, and subsequent episodes of symptomatic ventricular tachycardia, occurs more rapidly with exercise. Patients with ARC are counseled against participation in vigorous or competitive sports. Patients may present with pain, palpitations, syncope, and/or heart failure. Some will have an initial presentation of sudden cardiac death. The ECG of ARC has a distinctive epsilon wave and T wave inversions in leads V1-V3.

Wave, spin, last they know
Reroute retrograde blood flow
Pre-vertebral block
Use of arm near faint is key
History spells syncope

Subclavian Steal Syndrome

Subclavian steal syndrome results from a narrowing or blockage in a subclavian artery proximal to the takeoff of the vertebral artery. Vigorous arm use results in blood being siphoned retrograde from the vertebrobasilar circulation to supply the arm. Symptoms of subclavian steal syndrome include vertigo, syncope, and arm claudication.

Current takes a ride
Sprint sparks ventricles inside
Narrow QRS
Nodal paths: one fast, one slow
Adenosine, take straw, BLOW

Atrioventricular Node Reentrant Tachycardia

Atrioventricular Node Reentrant Tachycardia or AVNRT is the most common paroxysmal sustained narrow supraventricular tachycardia. In AVNRT, the AV node contains dual conduction pathways – one FAST to conduct and slow to repolarize, the other SLOW to conduct but fast to repolarize. A typical carousel circuit is started when a premature atrial contracted beat is conducted down the SLOW pathway and up the FAST. The ventricles are regularly and rapidly depolarized. The circuit can be broken by administration of adenosine or by vagal nerve stimulation, such as carotid massage or having the patient perform a Valsalva maneuver.

Heart inlet stretched full
No more space in pressured pool
Press liver and wait
Gush of blood to IVC
Flows past heart, fills JVP

Hepatojugular Reflex

The hepatojugular reflex is a physical exam finding consistent with a non-compliant right atrium. This may be due to right heart volume overload, right-sided heart failure, or restrictions on right heart forward flow, such as a large pulmonary embolism or cardiac tamponade. Pushing on the liver increases the venous return to the right heart from the inferior vena cava. If this blood is unable to spill into the right atrium, it will be pushed past the heart inlet up into the superior vena cava. The physical exam finding is a delayed rise in jugular vein volume following manual compression of the liver.

Painful leg dark blue
Venous blood gives limb its hue
Massive DVT
Lysis, declot, make it brisk
Full extremity at risk

Phlegmasia cerulea dolens

Phlegmasia cerulea dolens (PCD) is an inflamed blue painful leg due to extensive iliofemoral clot with compromise of arterial flow. Venous blood trapped in the leg gives it its cyanotic/blue hue. PCD is a life-threatening and limb-threatening condition. There is a high risk of gangrene and amputation of the leg if the clot is not quickly lysed and the vein recanalized.

Gelatinous blob
Tethered stalk, weaving bob
Nidus for blood clots
Diastolic tumor plop
Resect, emboli will stop

Cardiac Myxoma

Myxomas are the most common primary cardiac neoplasm. The typical myxoma is pedunculated and gelatinous in consistency. Approximately 80% originate in the left atrium and symptoms suggest mitral valve obstruction with the development of dyspnea, orthopnea, hemoptysis, and pulmonary edema. Patients often have constitutional symptoms of fever, weight loss. Physical exam may reveal a 'tumor plop.' Systemic embolization presents in about 25% of patients, most with neurologic signs. Cardiac surgical evaluation is indicated.

Crash! Arrives the cart
'We need to restart your heart!'
Startled. Brushing teeth.

ECG Artifact

ECG artifacts are electrocardiographic alterations, not related to cardiac activity, that are superimposed on the surface ECG. Examples include muscle movement from shivering, hiccups, brushing teeth and Parkinsonian tremor. The true spike structure and rate of the baseline ECG can often be divined through close examination of the trace and the use of calipers.

Giant silhouette
Pericardium beset
Heart takes laps in pool
Low voltage on ECG
Up down tracing swings gently

Pericardial Effusion with Electrical Alternans

Pericardial effusions may grow slowly over time to large proportions, allowing the heart to swing back and forth. The effect of this swinging on the surface electrocardiogram (ECG) is a beat-to-beat changing of axis, best seen on the rhythm strip, in a phenomenon called 'electrical alternans.' The effusion may also lead to muffling of the electrical signal, such that all leads show low voltage.

Ticking bloody bomb
Gentle exam, light, be calm
Thin-walled, stretched balloon
With each beat, less time to lose
Diagnose, deflate, defuse

Abdominal Aortic Aneurysm

Abdominal aortic aneurysm (AAA) is a potentially deadly complication of atherosclerotic changes to the distal aorta, most often below the level of the renal arteries. To be called an aneurysm, there must be a focal, full-thickness dilatation to more than 50% the normal diameter. Patients with an intact AAA may be asymptomatic or present with abdominal or back pain not related to a rupture. Diagnosis is made by specific imaging studies, such as ultrasound or CT. The risk of rupture usually exceeds the risk of repair when the AAA is >5.5cm. For smaller asymptomatic aneurysms, observation is recommended.

Idle hands may tug
Generator not held snug
Subtle spin with time
Loss of capture, first alarm
Paced phrenic, plexus of arm

Twiddler's Syndrome

Twiddler's syndrome is a complication of cardiac implantable electronic devices, such as pacemakers or implantable defibrillators, in which twisting of the pulse generator in its pocket results in lead dislodgement. Patients may present with symptoms related to bradyarrhythmias or to electrical pacing of the diaphragm or arm as the pacing leads are free to move within the chest.

Free wall stunned and lax
Furious apex contracts
Clot slams shut the door
RV echo key sign seen
Apex bouncing trampoline

McConnell's Sign

McConnell's sign, named for Michael V. McConnell MD, MSEE, is a distinct echocardiographic finding described in patients with acute pulmonary embolism. The echocardiogram shows right ventricular dysfunction with akinesia of the free wall but preserved motion at the apex. In McConnell's sign, the apex has been described as a trampoline bouncing up and down while the rest of the RV remains still.

Corset, narrow waist
Cinched below where knob is traced
3 sign, back ribs notched
BP above driven high
From low flow where kidneys lie

Aortic Coarctation

Aortic coarctation (AoC) is a congenital defect with a narrowed cinching of the aorta where the ductus arteriosus enters. On a plain chest film, the 'figure 3 sign' is formed by pre-stenotic dilatation of the aortic arch and left subclavian artery, the indentation at the coarctation site and post-stenotic dilatation of the descending aorta. A plain film may also show rib-notching due to collateral vessels connecting the superior arterial system to the lower body. With AoC, there is often secondary hypertension with the blood pressure higher in the upper than lower extremities. This hypertension is due to under-perfusion of the kidneys with subsequent release of vasoactive hormones and increased salt and water retention.

Nicotine or weed
Acral vessels scar and bead
Fingers, toes turn black
Young, male classic corkscrew wound
Smoking stopped, or digits pruned

Thromboangiitis Obliterans

Thromboangiitis obliterans, also known as Buerger's disease for Leo Buerger (1879-1943), is a disease of smokers, involving a progressive, inflammatory, occlusive, non-atherosclerotic vasculopathy of the hands and feet. There may also be ocular involvement with retinal artery occlusion. Patients are most often young (<40yo) and male, though the disease may be seen in older patients with cardiovascular risk factors. Buerger's disease presents with Raynaud's type demarcation of the fingers and toes, with progressive tissue ischemia. Angiography shows 'corkscrew collaterals.' The disease may progress to gangrene and autoamputation smoking continues.

Sudden painful shock
Leg's stopped inflow, rapid block
Pulseless, cool, numb, weak
Local plaque cracked, gone awry
Incoming large emboli

Acute Limb Ischemia

Acute limb ischemia may be due to in-situ thrombosis, arterial dissection, embolism, or trauma. Venous disease, such as the extensive deep vein thrombosis of phlegmasia cerulea dolens, can also lead to impaired arterial perfusion. The examination of an acutely ischemic limb is recalled by the six Ps: pain, poikilothermia, pallor, pulselessness, paresthesia and paralysis. Acute limb ischemia can threaten both loss of limb and life unless perfusion is rapidly restored. The reperfused limb is at risk for the development of compartment syndrome and rhabdomyolysis from injured muscles.

Arm day, lifting weights
Notice limb red, hand inflates
Ascends up the limb
One arm normal, one red hulk
DVT source of new bulk

Paget-Schroetter Syndrome

Paget-Schroetter Syndrome, named for Sir James Paget and Leopold Schroetter in 1949, is effort-induced deep vein thrombosis of an upper extremity. The result is a plethoric, edematous arm. Risk factors for the thrombosis include a subclavian vein compressed by anatomic structures, permanent pacemaker implantation, subclavian vein catheterization and the post-mastectomy syndrome. Most cases, though, are idiopathic. The proximal deep vein thrombosis is treated with thrombolysis and anticoagulation.

Sore throat, panicked look
Hot potato voice textbook
Straining in tripod
Neck film, thin air, plump thumb sign
Secured airway: aim divine

Acute Epiglottitis

Acute epiglottitis may be infectious or non-infectious. Hemophilus influenzae B infection was a common cause in the past but has been less so since the introduction of a vaccine. Caustic ingestion, thermal injury and trauma are all non-infectious etiologies. Epiglottitis leads to swelling of the supraglottic larynx and narrowing of the airway, with the 'thumb sign' on a lateral neck film denoting a swollen epiglottis. A 'hot potato' voice, the patient assuming a tripod position, and drooling are all signs of a threatened airway. Anesthesia evaluation is warranted.

Frantic, gulping breath
Tips balance from acid death
Metabolic mess
Heaving, hurling CO2
Raise pH of bitter stew

Kussmaul Breathing

Kussmaul breathing was described by Adolph Kussmaul (1822-1902), a German physician, poet, and student of Virchow. Kussmaul breathing is a breathing pattern in response to a severe metabolic acidosis, such as diabetic ketoacidosis. Kussmaul breathing, with repetitive, rapid, deep breaths, dramatically increases minute ventilation and, thus, reduces the partial pressure of carbon dioxide, pCO2. The resultant respiratory alkalosis balances the severe metabolic acidosis, bringing the body's pH closer to normal.

Film jet black one side
Lung down, vessels pushed aside
Blood flow slowly crushed
Needle intercostal hiss
Veins un-kinked, fatal near miss

Tension Pneumothorax

A tension pneumothorax occurs when the air around a collapsed lung is pressurized, typically from a ball-valve phenomenon, and the volume of air around the collapsed lung increases with each breath. This pressure pushes the mediastinum and opposite lung away from the collapsed lung, compressing the superior and inferior vena cavae. The tension pneumothorax's pressure must be released, typically by placing a large-bore needle into the second intercostal space on the side of the pneumothorax. Without this release, the patient will go into cardiovascular collapse.

Cool desperation
Sine waves of respiration
Central apneas
Rapid deep then slowing small
Repeat, repeat, that is all

Cheyne Stokes Respirations

Cheyne Stokes respirations, named for a 19th century description by John Cheyne and William Stokes, is a pattern of breathing which varies between two extremes: apnea and high tidal volume tachypnea. The cycling between these two patterns takes on a sine wave. Affected patients often have congestive heart failure or neurologic damage to their brain's respiratory center. The Cheyne Stokes pattern can be observed as a dying patient nears death.

Diaphragm pushed flat
Such altered mechanics that
Ribs suck in each breath
Blebbed, puffed, stretched lungs leave no room
Sides retract as by vacuum

Hoover Sign

The Hoover sign, named for Charles Franklin Hoover (1865-1927), refers to inspiratory retraction of the lower rib cage from severe chronic obstructive pulmonary disease (COPD). In COPD, there is a loss of lung elastic recoil and subsequent air-trapping. This leads to hyperinflation of the lungs and flattening of the diaphragms, which are anchored to the sides of the lower ribs. With inspiratory effort, the flattened diaphragms contract, pulling inward on the lower ribs, a paradoxical motion in inspiration.

Widespread mucus plugs
Hyphae encased sticky slugs
Eosinophils
Sudden uptick wheeze disease
Elevated IgEs

Allergic Bronchopulmonary Aspergillosis

Allergic Bronchopulmonary Aspergillosis (ABPA) is a pulmonary disease found in patients with long-standing asthma or those with cystic fibrosis. Their underlying disease is exacerbated due to an allergic reaction to colonizing *Aspergillus fumigatus,* resulting in thick, tenacious sputum production. Serologic testing shows increased levels of IgE to *A. fumigatus*. Radiology demonstrates mucus plugging, bronchiectasis and the 'finger in glove' sign of mucoid impaction. Treatment is directed at the allergic response, with prednisone, but may also include treatment of the colonizing *Aspergillus* with itraconazole.

Subtle loss of breath
Reduced GM-CSF
Signal for clean sweep
Alveoli clogged with gel
Crazy paving each air cell

Pulmonary Alveolar Proteinosis

Pulmonary alveolar proteinosis (PAP) is a lung disease characterized by the accumulation of amorphous, periodic acid-Schiff (PAS)-positive lipoproteinaceous material in the distal air spaces. The most common primary type of PAP in adults is due to autoantibodies against Granulocyte-Macrophage Colony-Stimulating Factor (GM-CSF). This factor is responsible for signaling alveolar macrophages to clear pulmonary surfactant. The typical age of PAP presentation is 40-50 years. Most patients are current or former cigarette smokers. Patients present with insidious onset of dyspnea. HRCT shows 'crazy-paving' polygonal shapes superimposed on ground glass. Treatment can involve whole lung lavage, inhaled GM-CSF, and, rarely, lung transplant.

Rib cage chunk cracked free
Chest, chunk move oppositely
Blunt trauma breaks loose
Breathing pattern doomed to fail
If not rapid repair flail

Flail Chest

Flail chest is due to multiple rib fractures which allow a segment of the chest to float freely. Flail chest is most commonly due to blunt trauma, such as a collision between the chest and a steering wheel, or an assault, as with a baseball bat. The chunk of chest wall is independent from the respiratory movement and moves opposite from the rest of the chest, e.g., out with exhalation and inward with inhalation. The paradoxical movement can compromise respiratory effort and may require intubation and ventilatory support. Thoracic surgical input is warranted.

Broken beating sweep
Can't clear mucus up from deep
Flaw since fetal life
Sidedness of organs skew
No beat, total switcheroo

Primary Ciliary Dyskinesia

Primary ciliary dyskinesia (PCD) is a genetic disease resulting in dysfunctional cilia. In the fetus, the reduction of cilia function may lead to a loss of 'sided-ness' to organ development and may result in a mirror image of the usual body anatomy, called situs inversus. Ciliary dysfunction in later life leads to chronic sinusitis and bronchiectasis. Both men and women with PCD have reduced or absent fertility due to poor motility of sperm and dysfunction of fallopian tube cilia, respectively.

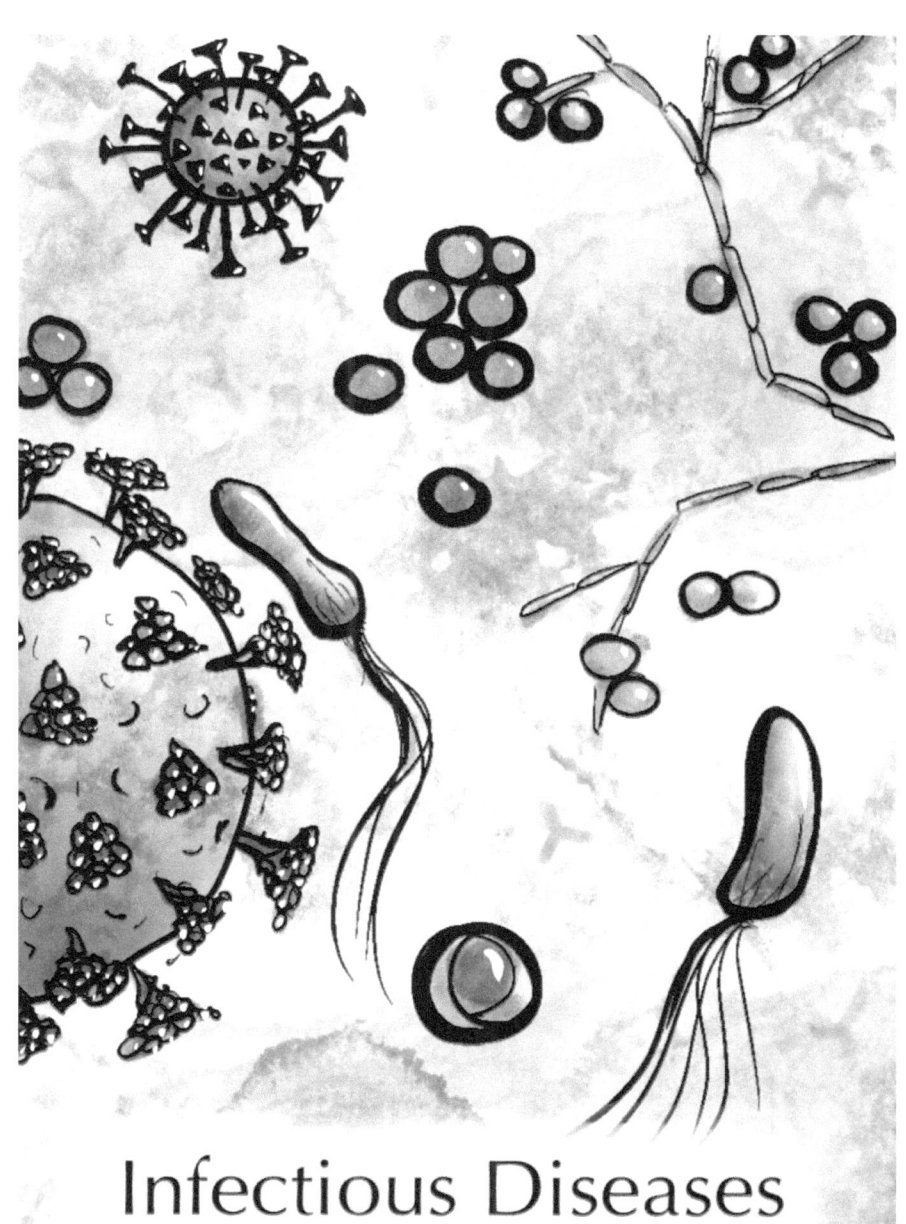
Infectious Diseases

Infectious Disease
Kanshen-Sho

World awash in pests
Wait chance to invade, infest
Suck life, spread anew

Pruned immunity
Neisseria M and *G*
Infect more, harm less
Defense weakened from end's lack
Weapons missing for attack

Terminal Complement Deficiency

Terminal complement deficiency is the absence of components C5-C9 in the complement cascade and results in an inability to form the membrane attack complex (MAC). Patients with this non-cellular immunodeficiency are susceptible to recurrent *Neisseria* infections, though these are typically milder and have a lower mortality rate. The immunological profile of terminal complement deficiency is normal C3 and C4 levels but a low CH50. Patients should receive vaccination against *Neisseria* infection.

Contact human skin
Larvae leave soil, burrow in
Find their way to lungs
Coughed up, swallowed, fertile worm
Steroids: overwhelmed with squirm

Strongyloides stercolis

Infectious larvae of *Strongyloides stercolis* are found in warm soil and can enter the skin through bare feet or through work with soil, e.g., construction workers or farmers. Human T-lymphotrophic virus-1 (HTLV-1) positivity increases the risk of co-infection. Larvae traverse a path through the lungs, where they may cause an eosinophilic Loffler's syndrome with cough and wheeze, on their way to the small intestines. The worms have a rapid lifecycle and auto-infection may occur when intestinal transit is slow. Treatment with steroids or immunosuppressant medications can trigger an overwhelming and potentially fatal hyperinfection.

Dust from valley winds
Inhaled barrel spores bore in
Spherules filled to burst
Fever, cough, skin, ankles, wrist
Treat for CAP, symptoms persist

Coccidioidomycosis

Coccidioidomycosis is also known as Valley fever. Barrel-shaped arthroconidia lie dormant in the soil of the Southwestern United States and may be aerosolized and inhaled. Once in the lungs, the fungus transforms into spherules. Infections are often asymptomatic, though they can present as community-acquired pneumonia (CAP) which does not respond to typical antibiotics. Extra-pulmonary manifestations include erythema nodosum, fatigue, and distal joint arthralgias referred to as 'desert rheumatism'. Infections can rarely spread hematogenously to the central nervous system and to vertebrae. Definitive treatment of coccidioidomycosis requires prolonged courses of anti-fungal therapy.

Death of spirochete
Whirling storm of rash, pain, heat
Bug's final hurrah
NSAID, steroid dose may quell
Woe to those who say or spell

Jarisch-Herxheimer Reaction

A Jarisch-Herxheimer (JH) reaction, named for Adolf Jarisch and Karl Herxheimer, is the difficult to spell and pronounce immunologic response to the deaths, usually by antibiotic treatment, of infecting spirochetes. The original description detailed fever and rash seen in patients receiving mercury treatment for syphilis. In their death throes, spirochetes release endotoxin which can sicken the host. The JH reaction can be limited by treatment with NSAIDs and steroids.

Late Summer Lake swim
Face splash, ingress comes at whim
Thin cribriform plate
LP gush gray CSF
Days rush fever, stupor, death

Primary amebic meningoencephalitis

Primary amebic meningoencephalitis is an acute hemorrhagic cerebral infection caused by *Naegleria fowleri*. The amoebae are found in warm fresh water and typically enter the CNS through the cribriform plate. Patients experience a rapid deterioration with progressive brain-swelling, coma and death, all within a mean timeframe of five days. Attempts to treat the infection have included combinations of Amphotericin B, fluconazole, rifampin, azithromycin and miltefosine, with very limited success.

Hours post picnic
Stem to stern GI tract sick
Rough spell, most well quick
Same bug: bloodstream, red cells burst
Rubbed in wound, gangrene's the worst

Clostridium perfringens

Perfringens is derived from Latin *per* ("through") and *frango* ("burst") referring to the bacteria's effect in disrupting tissue. *Clostridium perfringens* is a common cause of foodborne illness, typically presenting as vomiting and diarrhea that rapidly resolve. Bloodstream infections cause massive, often fatal hemolysis. Soft tissue and muscle infection results in gas gangrene, requiring prompt surgical debridement and systemic antibiotics.

Porcine tapeworm eggs
Hatch in gut and stretch their legs
Dot the CNS
Cloaked larvae spread at leisure
When revealed: swelling, seizure

Neurocysticercosis

Neurocysticercosis results from the ingestion of food contaminated with *Taenia solium* (pork tapeworm) eggs. Larvae hatch in the small intestines and migrate to a variety of tissues, including muscle, liver, brain, and eye. Cysts, comprised of a scolex with a bladder, evade the immune system and patients are often asymptomatic. Symptoms arise from mechanical disruption, e.g., cysts growing behind the eye, or when the larvae die and calcify, activating the immune system. Brain edema and inflammation, in response to dying cysts, is a major cause of secondary epilepsy in endemic parts of the world.

Caribbean jaunt
Bloodthirsty mosquitos taunt
Fever, diffuse rash
Crippling pain follows beach trip
Hand, wrist, ankle more than hip

Chikungunya

Chikungunya is carried by the Aedes mosquito. The infection spans a broad geography, which includes the Caribbean and Southeastern US. The name comes from the Makonde language and means 'that which bends up.' Symptoms include fever, rash, and severe joint pain, involving distal joints more than proximal. Joint pain can recur or become chronic. The pain may be intense and disabling. Rarely, patients may have additional severe complications, including respiratory failure, myocarditis, hepatitis, and acute flaccid paralysis. Infections are managed with supportive treatment.

Liquid pools in place
Poorly cleaned, drops sprayed at face
Fountains, old AC
Fever, cough, upset GI
Awful CAP, all gone awry

Legionnaires' Disease

Legionella Pneumonia or Legionnaires' Disease, named after the outbreak at the 1976 American Legion meeting, is a severe pulmonary infection occurring after exposure to water or soil contaminated with *Legionella*. Outbreaks cluster around contamination of water supplies at community sites such as hotels, apartment buildings, and shared pools. Patient risk factors include older age, smoking, and pre-existing lung, heart, or kidney disease. Clinical features common to *Legionella* pneumonia are gastrointestinal symptoms, liver enzyme elevation, hyponatremia, and failure to respond to beta-lactam antibiotic monotherapy. Treatment requires fluoroquinolones or macrolide antibiotics.

Worker from Brazil
Fever, lymph nodes, feeling ill
Weeks of small pustules
Vertigo, gait thrown off keel
Path shows budding pilot's wheel

Paracoccidioidomycosis

Paracoccidioidomycosis is a systemic mycotic disease endemic to South America, with most infections occurring in Brazil. Men are infected more often than women and the infection has been associated with alcoholism, smoking and outdoor occupations, such as farming or construction. Symptoms range from asymptomatic to acute, subacute, and chronic forms. Symptomatic patients often present with prominent lymph nodes, liver, spleen and bone marrow involvement, gingival 'mulberry' lesions, and pulmonary disease. The yeast form of the fungus takes the shape of a budding 'ship's wheel' or 'pilot's wheel.'

Hands feet numb, gait slow
Sushi eaten long ago
Bizarre neutrophils
Stolen B12 for own fuel
Large knobbed lidded eggs in stool

B12 Deficiency from Fish Tapeworm

Dibothriocephalus latus, also known as *Diphyllobothrium latum*, is a fish tapeworm. It is the largest tapeworm that can infect people, growing up to 30 feet long. Infection comes from eating raw infected freshwater predator fish, such as pike and trout. Adult worms develop in the intestines and can cause mechanical blockages. The worms also suck on the intestinal wall and compete for vitamin B12 absorption. This competition can lead to B12 deficiency and subsequent neurologic and hematologic manifestations. Diagnosis of *D. latus* infection is made through discovery of distinctive large knobbed lidded eggs in the stool. Infections are treated with praziquantel.

'Mono' gets more press
Raw colitis when suppressed
Many calling cards
Dark blue owl's eyes set apart
Ganciclovir, urgent start

Cytomegalovirus Infection

Cytomegalovirus or CMV typically causes a mild febrile illness in immunocompetent adults. Severe infection occurs in immunosuppressed hosts with manifestations including hemorrhagic colitis, retinitis, pneumonitis, and meningitis. Biopsies of involved tissues show characteristic basophilic 'Owl's Eye' inclusions. Patients with prolonged immunosuppression, e.g., transplant patients, should receive CMV prophylaxis. Treatment of CMV infections can include ganciclovir or foscarnet.

Fresh air, mountain streams
Water not clean as it seems
Weeks on symptoms start
Cramping, loose stool, scare for host
Haunting wide-eyed floating ghosts

Giardia Infection

The trophozoite form of the protozoan parasite *Giardia lamblia* or *duodenalis* resembles 'angry old men' or ghosts. The parasite infects the proximal small bowel epithelia following ingestion of cysts, typically from contaminated water. Patients may be asymptomatic, or they can have acute watery, fatty diarrhea and/or develop chronic malabsorption. Diagnosis is made through antigen detection or stool microscopy. *Giardia* can be treated with either tinidazole or metronidazole.

Safari nightmare
Firm wounds, now larvae in there
Skin actually crawls
Reach in, fish out, wriggling snot
Drop, lose track, perish the thought

Cutaneous myiasis

Cutaneous myiasis due to infestation by larvae of *Cordylobia anthopophagia*, also called the Tumbu or Mango fly. The fly lays eggs under the skin during a bite. Patients present with multiple wiggling sinuses containing fly larvae. Extraction is eased by first suffocating the larvae with petroleum jelly. Patients may require antibiotics for any surrounding cellulitis.

Safari brought home
Pics of blue skies, herds that roam
Painful black chancre
Fever, jaundice, shaking chills
Fly bites transmit grievous ills

Trypanosomiasis

Trypanosoma brucei, rhodesiense (East) is rarer and more fulminant than the *gambiense* (West) strain of African Sleeping Sickness. A chancre forms at the site of a bite from an infected Tsetse fly. Several weeks later, the infected patient develops high fevers, rigors, jaundice and disseminated intravascular coagulation. Infections with the *rhodesiense* strain of *Trypanosoma brucei* are often fatal before the patient develops the chronic encephalitis picture known as 'sleeping sickness.' The treatment regimen hinges on the degree of involvement of the central nervous system and requires a lumbar puncture for stratification.

Liver's lily cyst
Hooklets, daughters swirl like mist
Expansive dark pond
Albendazole, sharp dissect
Puncture, aspirate, inject

Hydatid Cyst Disease

Echinococcus granulosus is the dog tapeworm which can cause systemic cystic disease when eggs are ingested by humans, its accidental host. Liver involvement is common and often asymptomatic, with symptoms depending on the size and location of cysts. Cysts may become symptomatic when they rupture, e.g., causing biliary obstruction, peritonitis, portal hypertension, and/or anaphylaxis. Diagnosis is made through ultrasound showing complex cysts with hydatid sand or features such as the 'water lily sign' with detachment of the endocyst membrane floating free within the pericyst. Treatment includes albendazole, surgery and PAIR (puncture, aspirate, instillation, and re-aspiration).

Beach, hand cut on shell
Within hours, temp, unwell
Bloody, tense bullae
Underlying cirrhosis
Paves a path for necrosis

Vibrio Necrotizing Fasciitis

Vibrio vulnificus is a Gram-negative curved bacillus of the family Vibrionaceae. The bacteria thrive in warm temperatures and brackish water. When wounds are exposed to contaminated water, *Vibrio* can cause necrotizing skin infections with bullae, resembling gas gangrene. Such infections require immediate surgical debridement and systemic antibiotics. Patients may also develop primary septicemia through the consumption of contaminated raw or undercooked seafood. Patients with immunocompromising conditions, including chronic liver disease, iron-overload, and cancer, are at increased risk of complications.

Beach, covered with bites
Painless ulcers dot bite sites
Plump base underneath
Full thickness shows clustered cells
Cultured, long whip is bug's tell

Cutaneous Leishmaniasis

Leishmania species are transmitted by sandflies and are the agents of leishmaniasis. Leishmaniasis has three pathologic forms: cutaneous, mucocutaneous, and visceral, also known as kala azar. The cutaneous variant is most common and is characterized by papules that ulcerate at the site of the fly bite. Biopsy shows host macrophages enveloping amastigotes. Culture allows for growth of the parasite to the promastigote stage, which is distinctive for the whip emanating from one pole.

Eggs go down the hatch
Through gut, portal vein will catch
Liver to riled lungs
Coughed up, swallowed, worms mature
Zillion eggs, species secure

Ascariasis

Ascaris lumbricoides is a round worm gastrointestinal parasite which has a complicated lifecycle. Eggs are ingested in contaminated food and hatch in the small intestines. Larvae then travel to the lungs, before being coughed up and swallowed back into the GI tract. A mature female worm expels 200,000 eggs a day. Most infections are asymptomatic, though there may be pulmonary symptoms of cough and wheeze during larval transit. Adult worms may cause obstructive symptoms within the intestines and shocked surprise when they exit through the rectum, mouth, or nose.

Fused lymphatic blight
Years out from mosquito bite
Form elephantine
Filariae cause lymph duct scar
Leg takes on shape of Babar

Filariasis

Wucheria bancrofti is one of three roundworms which cause filariasis and elephantiasis. The organism is spread by mosquito bite and has a long-life cycle with adult worms finally migrating to the lymph system. The quantity of adult worms, the immune system and secondary bacterial infections all determine the eventual outcome of the parasitic infection. Some, but not all, infections will lead to permanent disability from grossly disfigured limbs with thickened, hardened skin.

From roses, rosettes
Creeping vine of fungal threat
Trails from thorn's sharp prick
Buds entice, inhale sweet bloom
Weak lungs, though, may breathe in doom

Sporotrichosis

Sporotrichosis is caused by *Sporothrix schenckii*, often called rose-handlers' disease. The fungus, notable for rosette-shaped conidia, is implanted from the soil into the skin through contact of a small wound, e.g., a thorn prick. Subcutaneous nodules, often painless, extend up the limb via the lymph system and may ulcerate and discharge pus. Inhalation of the fungus by patients with underlying pulmonary disease, such as chronic obstructive pulmonary disease, can result in a severe fungal pneumonia. The most common treatment of sporotrichosis is months of oral itraconazole.

Light sprinkling of snow
Scrape the tongue, dark red below
White scourge of young mouths
Lost, suppressed, altered flora
Portal for yeast plethora

Thrush

Oral candidiasis or thrush is a common yeast infection of the mouth. Risk factors include infancy or old age, underlying immunodeficiency, dry mouth, smoking, broad-spectrum antibiotics, and inhaled corticosteroids used to treat pulmonary diseases. Oral *Candida* infection presents as a white coating on the tongue which easily scrapes off to reveal an erythematous base. Clotrimazole troches, among other therapies, are effective at treating thrush.

Heaped up flesh gone numb
Bugs clip cool nerves one by one
High count bacilli
Laissez faire immune offline
Leads to facies leonine

Leprosy

Leprosy, or Hansen's disease for Gerhard Hansen (1841-1912), is an infection caused by the slow-growing bacteria, *Mycobacterium leprae*. The extent of infection is dependent upon the host's immune response. A 'lepromatous' response results in a high bacteria count and overwhelming infection. *M. leprae* grow best at 27-33 degree Celsius and tend to infect the cooler areas of the body, including nerves, skin, eyes, the lining of the nose, and the tips of hands and feet. Extensive involvement of the skin of the face results in a leonine, or lion-like, face.

Spotty crops frustrate
Small nodules umbilicate
Spread from skin-to-skin
Scratch autoinoculates
Liquid nitrogen ablates

Molluscum contagiosum

Molluscum contagiosum, caused by a DNA poxvirus, are spread by fomites, autoinoculation, and skin-to-skin contact. Swimmers may acquire the infection through exposure in contaminated public pools. Molluscum present as multiple, small, flesh-colored, dome-shaped papules with central umbilication. Treatment often involves cryoablation with liquid nitrogen.

Dappled dark with pale
Light scraping from skin's fine scale
Micro pasta dish
To be sure cure endures
Azole or dandruff tinctures

Pityriasis versicolor

Pityriasis versicolor, a skin condition of hypo- and hyperpigmentation, is due to infection with the fungus *Malassezia furfur*. Scrapings of affected skin look like 'spaghetti and meatballs' under light microscopy. Pityriasis versicolor is treated with topical selenium sulfide, ketoconazole shampoo or oral itraconazole.

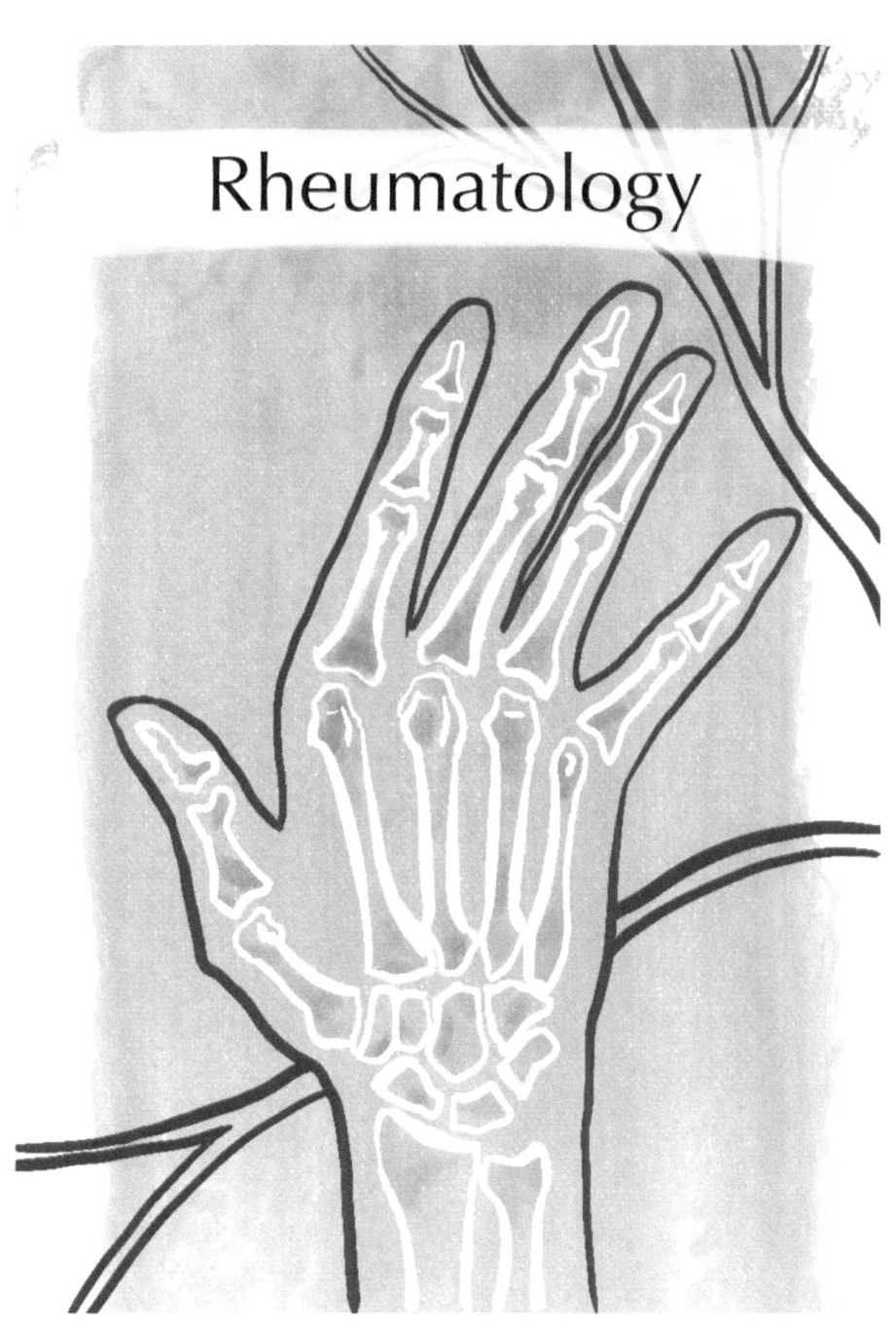

Rheumatology

Rheumatology
Riumachigaku

Fires burnt, hot or cold
Pain, anguish, a tale foretold
Ambush from within

Puffy hands stretched taut
Fatigued, pale, lips thin, distraught
Dark black sticky stools
NPO for EGD
Best guess what GI might see?

Gastric Antral Vascular Ectasia

Gastric antral vascular ectasia (GAVE) is a source of GI bleeding in both limited and diffuse systemic sclerosis. Endoscopy shows the typical findings of 'watermelon stomach' with red stripes radiating from the pylorus. The connection between systemic sclerosis and GAVE is not well understood, though GAVE is often more severe in early diffuse systemic sclerosis and appears to improve with immunosuppression.

Seared muscles grow weak
Syndrome's rapid blazes wreak
Steel wool scars on lungs
Real mechanics' hands less rough
Lab predicts lung fate that's tough

Antisynthetase Syndrome

Antisynthetase syndrome is a rapidly progressive inflammatory myopathy. Patients may have features of fibrotic interstitial lung disease, small joint symmetric polyarthritis, Raynaud's phenomenon, and thick, cracked 'mechanics' hands.' The syndrome shares features of dermatomyositis. Anti-tRNA synthetase enzymes, including anti-Jo-1, correlate with poor interstitial lung disease outcomes.

Hives, sore joints flare out
Fever, chills, recurrent bouts
Hearing grows more faint
Cryopyrin from parent
Clogged tissues, proteins errant

Muckle-Wells Syndrome

Muckle-Wells Syndrome is a rare autosomal-dominant autoinflammatory disorder in the family of cryopyrin-associated periodic syndromes (CAPS). Cryopyrin is important in innate immunity as part of the multiprotein inflammasome. *NLRP3* is the mutated gene. Patients present with recurrent hives, small joint pain, fever, chills, and progressive hearing loss, as well as elevated C-reactive protein and amyloid A. With repeated bouts of inflammation, patients can develop AA amyloidosis. Treatment consists of IL-1 antagonists.

Shins splotched, purple red
Weakness, barely rise from bed
Joints achy and sore
Viral spree of HCV
Founts frosty immunity

Meltzer's Triad of Mixed Cryoglobulinemia

Meltzer's triad of mixed cryoglobulinemia:
1) palpable purpura from cutaneous vasculitis; 2) arthralgias; and 3) weakness from peripheral neuropathy. Hepatitis C infection has been reported in a high percentage of mixed cryoglobulinemia cases. Other etiologies include autoimmune disease, such as Systemic Lupus Erythematosus (SLE) and Sjogren's disease, and lymphoproliferative disorders. The kidneys may be involved with a membranoproliferative glomerulonephritis pattern.

Inflamed MCPs
Crippling torching of both knees
Joints burled, bent and gnarled
Right treatment can obviate
Drug of choice methotrexate

Rheumatoid Arthritis

Rheumatoid arthritis (RA) primarily involves synovial joints and is a chronic, systemic, inflammatory, autoimmune disorder of unclear etiology. RA typically presents as polyarticular arthritis with an insidious onset of pain, stiffness and swelling of involved joints. The metacarpophalangeal and proximal interphalangeal joints of the hands, the wrists and the metatarsophalangeal joints of the toes are often affected. Morning stiffness is a prominent feature. Involvement of extraarticular organs, such as the eyes or lungs, occur in almost half of patients. Disease-modifying anti-rheumatic drug (DMARD) therapy, such as methotrexate, and tight control of flares have significantly improved outcomes for patients with RA.

Urate synthesis
Blocked with constant dose of this
Gout, stones, TLS
Rarely burns as if from sun
Avoid B*58:01

Allopurinol

Allopurinol is a xanthine oxidase inhibitor regularly used in the treatment and prophylaxis of gout and uric acid stones. It is also used in the prophylaxis of tumor lysis syndrome. This drug is associated with severe cutaneous adverse reactions (SCAR) in those with HLA*B58:01, typically Han Chinese, Thai, Korean and African populations. Concurrent diuretics, especially thiazides, and advanced renal insufficiency are also major risk factors for SCAR. Clinicians should test for the allele prior to prescribing allopurinol.

Ulcers of all lips
Pustule at prick of pin tips
Scourge of the Silk Road
Blinding blurring of both eyes
Vasculitis every size

Behcet Syndrome

Behcet Syndrome, named for Hulusi Behcet (1889-1948), a Turkish dermatologist, is an autoimmune disease known for recurrent oral and genital ulceration. Patients show pathergy, e.g., a pustule in response to a pin prick. The disease has broad clinical manifestations including uveitis, meningcencephalitis, pericarditis, arthritis, GI ulceraticns and small to large vessel vasculitis. The highest incidence of the disease is found in populations stemming from along the Ancient Silk Road.

Demarcation clear
Palms flushed there, pale fingers here
Blanched, numbed by the cold
Chilly change often benign
Tip necrosis a bad sign

Raynaud's Phenomenon

Raynaud's phenomenon, named for Auguste Gabriel Maurice Raynaud (1834-1881), is a vasospastic disorder affecting the small arteries of the fingers and toes in response to exposure to cold temperature. Rarely, the nose, ears, or lips may be affected. Distal to the vasospasm, the digit turns white and then blue, often with numbness or pain. As blood returns, the affected part turns red and often has a burning sensation. Secondary Raynaud's is associated with underlying diseases including hypothyroidism, autoimmune disease, hematologic disorders such as cryoglobulinemia, and mechanical injury or frostbite.

Tough to rise from bed
Rapid rate of red cell sed
Lazarus post pred
Lurking specter giant cell
Low bar to eval as well

Polymya gia Rheumatica

Polymya gia rheumatica is an inflammatory disorder affecting older (>50yo) patients and is characterized by morning shoulder and hip girdle stiffness, high inflammatory markers, and rapid clinical improvement with low-dose steroids. PMR can overlap with the more serious and morbid temporal arteritis, also known as giant cell arteritis or GCA. Patients diagnosed with PMR should be evaluated for signs and symptoms of GCA.

Curved fingers blanch white
Spiders flush, food sticks post bite
SubQ calcium
Thick tight skin of hands, feet, face
Mortal risk: pressured airspace

Limited Cutaneous Systemic Sclerosis

CREST, the acronym for calcinosis, Raynaud's, esophageal dysmotility, sclerodactyly and telangiectasias, has been renamed as limited cutaneous systemic sclerosis. Patients may present with some or all the CREST elements and are also at risk for morbid pulmonary hypertension. The autoantibodies anti-centromere and anti-SCL-70 are closely associated with this presentation.

Frostbite without cold
White count reduced manifold
Anti-helminthic
Cocaine cut to increase weight
Cuts the high and maims drug mate

Levamisole

Levamisole is an anti-helminthic drug used in the treatment of ascariasis and hookworm infections. Cocaine is regularly cut with the drug to increase its weight. Levamisole is associated with anti-neutrophil cytoplasmic antibody (ANCA) vasculitis, which can cause gangrenous skin lesions of acral skin, such as the nose, ear helices, fingers, and toes. The drug also causes leukopenia with increased risk of infection.

Flaming mid branches
Beaded flow, tissue blanches
Fibrinoid cell death
Rise in BP, GI vexed
Livedo, M multiplex

Polyarteritis Nodosa

Polyarteritis nodosa (PAN), a vasculitis of muscular medium- and small-sized arteries, has been associated with Hepatitis B infection, though less so with increasing rates of vaccination. Most cases are now idiopathic. PAN can affect almost any organ, with the kidneys, skin, joints, muscle, nerves, and gastrointestinal tract most often involved. The lungs are consistently spared. The inflammation of PAN is segmental, leading to a beaded appearance to affected arteries. Pathology shows transmural, homogenous fibrinoid necrosis with infiltrates of polymorphonuclear cells.

Often inflames knee
Rhomboids glint positively
Crown around the dens
Calcium in joint is seen
Flares managed by colchicine

Pseudogout

Pseudogout is inflammation due to the deposition of calcium pyrophosphate crystals (CPPD). Affected joints include the knees, usually the first joint affected, toes, wrists, shoulders, and ankles. Involvement around the second vertebra (C2) is known as the crowned dens syndrome. Radiologic features include chondrocalcinosis and calcification of the articular cartilage menisci. Crystals are rhomboid-shaped and weak positively birefringent. Treatment of pseudogout flares includes NSAIDs, colchicine and corticosteroid joint injection.

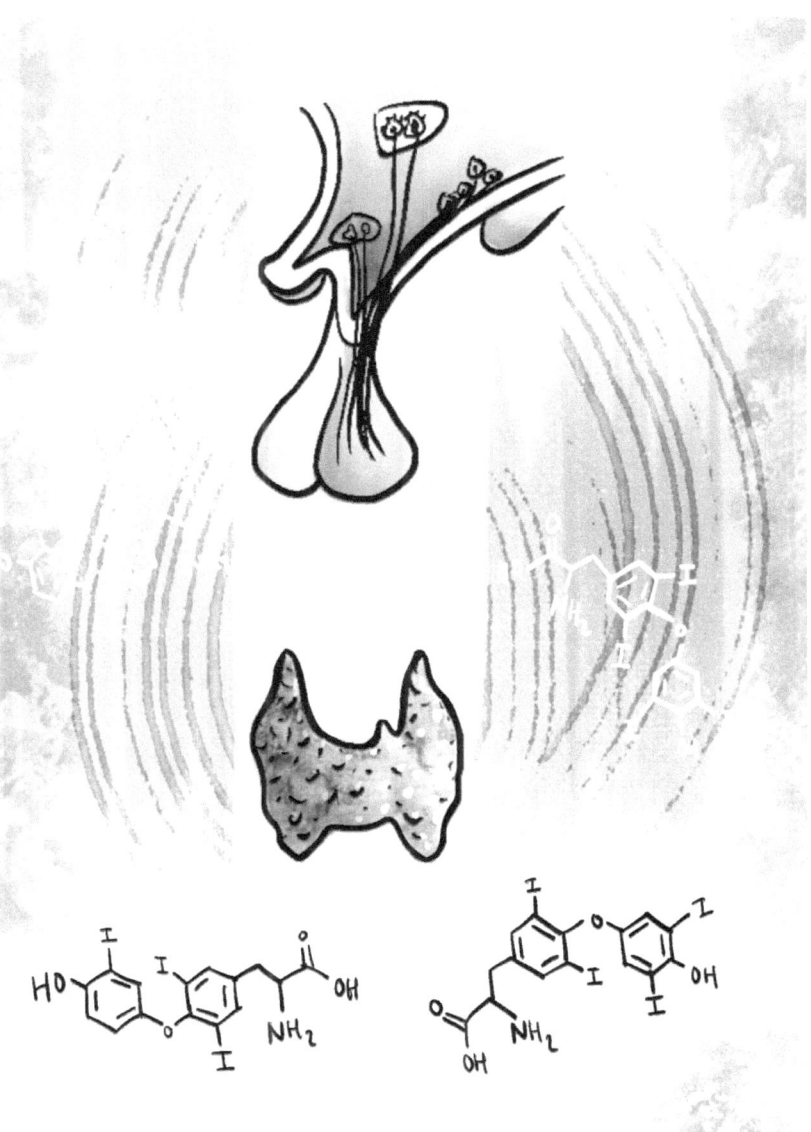

Endocrinology

Endocrinology
Naibunpitsu

Vital messaging
Commands, feedback, all take wing
Local or flung wide

Stress throws out of gear
Glucose up in stratosphere
And yet no ketones
Water loss drives thirst to drink
Kidneys wilt while brain cells shrink

Hyperosmolar Hyperglycemic State

Hyperosmolar hyperglycemic state is an endocrine emergency. Patients with Type II Diabetes Mellitus develop extreme hyperglycemia in response to a stressor, e.g., an infection, a myocardial infarction, or non-adherence to medication. This stressor results in gluconeogenesis, glycogenolysis and increased insulin resistance. The resulting hyperosmotic state leads to osmotic diuresis and volume depletion, osmotic shifts, and brain dehydration, with subsequent altered mental status, confusion, and coma. Patients often develop an acute kidney injury. Treatment includes volume resuscitation, free water replacement and insulin.

Berry bush, stung by bee
Chain reaction IgE
Mast cells detonate
Lips, tongue swell like ripe red fruits
Flush, faint, blood redistributes

Hymenoptera Venom Anaphylaxis

An anaphylactic reaction occurs with 0.3-3% of stings. The sting sets into motion IgE activation of mast cells and basophils. The subsequent chain reaction results in an exponential release of histamine and other vasoactive mediators. These mediators lead to urticaria, angioedema, including edema of the lips and airway, and ultimately, distributive shock.

Forced flood iodine
Swamps the works, a brief decline
Quick break in the storm

Wolff Chaikoff Effect

The Wolff Chaikoff effect is named for Jan Wolff and Israel Chaikoff. Iodine organification and both the formation and release of thyroid hormone are inhibited after a large dose of iodine. This effect is utilized in the treatment of thyroid storm and as preoperative preparation for thyroidectomy in Graves' disease. The effect forms the basis for the anti-thyroid cancer protective effect of high dose potassium iodide ingestion in the event of a radiation accident or nuclear weapon attack.

Late teens, Tanner 1
Sense of smell tests dull or none
Missing midline pulse

Kallmann Syndrome

Kallmann syndrome, named for the German-American geneticist Franz Josef Kallmann (1897-1965), is a form of hypothalamic hypogonadism with hypo- or anosmia. The syndrome results from the failure of neurons, both olfactory neurons and those responsible for Gonadotropin Releasing Hormone (GnRH) pulsatile release, to migrate through the olfactory placode during embryonic life. Males are more often affected than females. Patients present in their late teens with absent secondary sexual development. Patients may also have midline craniofacial defects such as cleft palate or coloboma.

Young man, growing thinner
Starved, chowing rice for dinner
Collapse, legs so weak
Goiter, moist skin, jittery
U waves splay on ECG

Thyrotoxic Periodic Paralysis

Thyrotoxic periodic paralysis results from sensitization of the sodium/potassium ATPase exchanger by the thyrotoxic state. Patients develop severe hypokalemia either after exercise due to high beta-adrenergic catecholamines, or after high carbohydrate meals, in response to insulin. The disorder is not familial though the population most affected is young East Asian men. The syndrome is treated by potassium supplementation, beta-blockade, and treating the underlying hyperthyroidism until the patient is euthyroid.

Mini mighty glands
Hide out beneath thyroid's span
Fine tune calcium
One (or four) goes on the fritz
Stones, groans, bones crumble to bits

Primary Hyperparathyroidism

Primary hyperparathyroidism, either due to an adenoma or hyperplasia, results in hypercalcemia, hypophosphatemia, and elevated urine calcium in the setting of an elevated or inappropriately normal parathyroid hormone (PTH) level. Hyperplasia of the four glands raises suspicion for an underlying genetic disorder, e.g., Multiple Endocrine Neoplasia 1. Patients with hyperparathyroidism may be asymptomatic or have wide-ranging symptoms including bone pain, kidney stones, constipation, and depression. Surgery is often the best management choice for patients who are symptomatic.

Thick, dark, velvet, lush
Scarf wraps neck, axilla plush
Hidden malady
Ineffective insulin
Rare a cancer grows within

Acanthosis Nigricans

Acanthosis nigricans is a dermatologic finding with hyperpigmented, velvety plaques primarily situated around the neck and in the axillae. They are associated with insulin resistance and are also seen in obesity, Type II diabetes mellitus, polycystic ovarian syndrome, and metabolic syndrome. Rarely, the plaques can be a sign of underlying malignancy, typically gastrointestinal adenocarcinomas.

Flush, sick after dish
Poorly stored plate dark meat fish
Spicy on palate
Within hour hits histamine
GI distress, ugly scene

Scombroid Fish Poisoning

The flesh of dark meat fish, including tuna, mackerel, and herring, contains high amounts of histidine. With inadequate refrigeration, bacteria convert histidine to histamine. The spoiled fish can have a 'peppery' flavor when ingested. Within one to two hours, patients develop flushing, sweating, urticaria, headache and diarrhea. Severe reactions include angioedema, respiratory arrest, cardiac arrest, and death.

Strong thirst cannot sate
Cells near saddle's morbid fate
Polyuria
Urine osm next to nil
DDAVP stems spill

Central Diabetes Insipidus

Central diabetes insipidus (CDI) results from either hypothalamic infiltration, such as from sarcoidosis or Langerhans cell histiocytosis, or from injury to the infundibular stalk or posterior pituitary. In the absence of anti-diuretic hormone (ADH), the kidneys are unable to concentrate urine. Patients present with hypotonic polyuria and polydipsia. With administration of 1-deamino-8-D-arginine vasopressin, also known as desmopressin or DDAVP, and an analogue of ADH, the kidney's tubules concentrate urine, distinguishing CDI from nephrogenic diabetes insipidus.

Iceberg near inlet
Arms down, blood squeaks by and yet
Arms up, cork! Flow squished
Eyes bulge, face swells, hard to breathe
Large goiter blocks SVC

Pemberton's Sign

Pemberton's Sign, named for Hugh Pemberton (1890-1956), detects venous obstruction in patients with thyroid goiters. The sign is positive when bilateral arm elevation causes facial plethora. This finding is attributed to a 'cork effect' with the goiter blocking the thoracic inlet and obstructing venous outflow from the head.

Puffy eyes, pulse low
Tendon strike: fast up, down slow
Tip toes stuck on pointe

Woltman's Sign

Woltman's sign, named for Henry Woltman (1889-1964) is the delayed relaxation of deep tendon reflexes in the setting of severe hypothyroidism. Reflexes have a normal brisk upstroke but then are 'hung up,' relaxing slowly back to neutral. This is best demonstrated in the Achilles tendon reflex. The delay in relaxation time appears to be proportional to the level of thyroid hormone deficiency. Differential diagnosis includes anorexia nervosa, advanced age, and beta-blocker use.

ACTH source
Wraps the bronchus, makes voice hoarse
Grows a buffalo
Thin arms, striped girth, face a moon
Occult mass un-occult soon

Paraneoplastic Cushing's Syndrome

Paraneoplastic Cushing's syndrome due to small cell lung cancer (SCLC) secreting adrenocorticotrophic hormone (ACTH). The poem describes features of hypercortisolemia with central obesity, dorsal fat pad also known as a 'buffalo hump,' and roundness and plethora of the face. The SCLC has become clinically apparent through both local effects on the recurrent laryngeal nerve and paraneoplastic ACTH production.

Gastroenterology & Hepatology

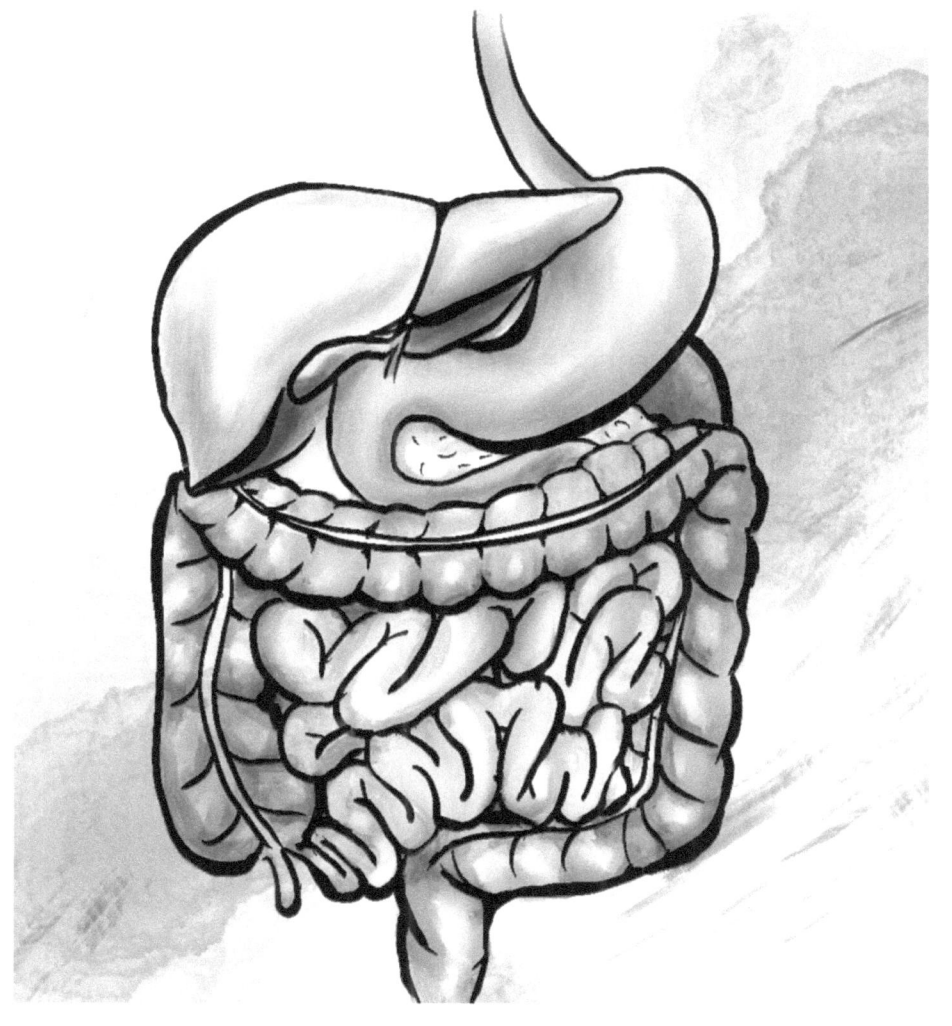

Gastroenterology/Hepatology
Icho Kanzo

Rejoice, feast and feed
System takes just what it needs
Refuse left behind

Baguette allergy
Blunted villi, atrophy
Anti-tTG
Iron slides by gut streamlined
Dermatitis serpentine

Celiac Disease

Celiac disease is the manifestation of an allergy to gluten. The disease has complex genetics and is linked to other autoimmune disorders. There is variable worldwide prevalence. The immune response results in blunting of the small intestine villi and malabsorption (notably of iron). Patients may be asymptomatic or have GI symptoms of diarrhea, abdominal pain, and bloating. Extraintestinal symptoms include the pruritic rash known as dermatitis herpetiformis, bone disease and peripheral neuropathies.

Foraging, fun day
Mushroom pizza, Cabernet
Liver liquifies

Amatoxin-Containing Mushroom Poisoning

Watery or bloody diarrhea develops within about seven hours of ingestion of an amatoxin-containing mushroom, such as *Amanita phylloides*, also known as the 'Death Cap' mushroom. This is followed by delayed massive liver necrosis, kidney failure, and disseminated intravascular coagulation. Treatment with IV silibinin or high dose IV penicillin G have been employed to reverse the toxic process, though with limited success. Amatoxin-induced liver failure has a high mortality rate, and many patients will die or require urgent liver transplantation.

Bloody nest of worms
Out from liver stream and squirm
Seeking better course
Wider, thinner, burst blood bath
Band, ablate, flow finds new path

Esophageal Varices

Esophageal varices are portosystemic shunts which open due to portal hypertension. The risk of variceal bleeding increases with enlarging radius of the varix. Treatment options range from non-selective beta-blockade to variceal banding to portal decompression with a TIPS (transjugular intrahepatic portosystemic shunt) procedure.

Endoscopic view
Misplaced vessel poking through
Only fools forget
Pumping stomach fundal bleed
Scope now, need of urgent speed

Dieulafoy Lesion

A Dieulafoy lesion, named for the French surgeon Paul Georges Dieulafoy (1839-1911), is an aberrant, dilated, submucosal gastric arteriole. It is typically found in the upper stomach on the lesser curvature. The artery may spontaneously bleed with arterial force, presenting dramatically. This upper gastrointestinal bleed requires immediate endoscopy and hemostatic intervention.

Firm ball liver's edge
Ducts' conflux in need of dredge
Inflates, filled with bile
Waste pigment spreads without pain
Due to slow loss of its drain

Courvoisier's Sign

Courvoisier's sign or law, named for the Swiss surgeon Ludwig Courvoisier (1843-1918), is a palpable gallbladder. The law states that this finding, without pain, in a jaundiced patient is consistent with malignant biliary obstruction. The malignancies most often associated with Courvoisier's sign are primary biliary or pancreatic in etiology.

Haustral sweep's slow swell
Borborygmi's loss a tell
Something's very wrong
Quiet before crisis stage
Call to Surgery: STAT page

Toxic Megacolon

Toxic megacolon results from progressive colonic dilatation and paralysis due to uncontrolled inflammation. Etiologies include inflammatory bowel disease and infection, e.g., *Clostridium difficile*. Patients present with systemic toxicity and a quiet abdominal exam. Imaging shows the colonic diameter >6cm. Urgent surgical evaluation is indicated, as is bowel rest and broad-spectrum antibiotics.

Weak spot back of throat
Outpouching in muscle coat
Pain, cough, hard to eat
Food gets stuck, fermenting slosh
Putrid breath defeats mouthwash

Zenker's Diverticulum

Zenker's diverticulum, named for Friedrich von Zenker (1825-1898), is a false diverticulum which protrudes through Killian's triangle between the thyropharyngeal and cricopharyngeal muscles. This pouch in the back of the throat can retain food, pills, and mucus, all which fester and cause bad breath. Patients may also complain of a gurgling sensation in their neck and dysphagia with swallowing. Typical patients are elderly men.

Cystic stone can't pass
Blocks common with inflamed mass
Fever, jaundice, pain
Release requires surgery
Cystic out, leave common free

Mirizzi Syndrome

Mirizzi syndrome, named for Argentinian surgeon Pablo Luis Mirizzi (1893-1964), is common hepatic duct obstruction caused by extrinsic compression from an impacted gallstone either in the cystic duct or at the infundibulum of the gallbladder. Compression of the common duct leads to cholestasis and can present as cholangitis. Surgical extraction with removal of the gallbladder and reconstruction of the common duct is indicated. There is an association with cholangiocarcinoma.

Snakes of gorgon writhe
Spreading out and to the side
Portocaval shunts
Fetal vein popped open thus
Knobby arms of octopus

Caput Medusae

Caput medusae or Medusa's head is a physical exam finding resembling the snakes of the mythical Gorgon. The umbilical vein is recanalized due to elevated portal pressure and connects to engorged superficial epigastric veins radiating out from the umbilicus.

Sternum, strong squeeze behind
Esophagus lost its mind
Trace of triple Lutz
Food can barely skate its course
Tube twisted by corkscrew force

Diffuse Esophageal Spasm

Diffuse esophageal spasm (DES) is a cause of dysphagia to both solids and liquids, and retrosternal, non-cardiac chest pain. The esophagus loses its controlled swallow-triggered wave and becomes spastic and irregular in its contractions. Barium swallow studies reveal a 'corkscrew' or 'rosary bead' appearance. Diagnosis is made through endoscopy plus/minus a manometry study. Therapy for DES includes controlling gastroesophageal reflux, proton pump inhibitors, peppermint oil, calcium channel blockers and botulinum toxin injections.

Gloved finger, much lube
Gently stretch the puckered tube
Swish from side to side
Up close care, surely accrues
Patient, nurses' love for you

Manual Disimpaction

In severe constipation, a hard stool ball can form in the rectum, resistant to chemical dissolution by either enema or laxatives. Manual fragmentation of the ball with a gloved and lubricated finger allows for passage of smaller fecal pieces and provides significant relief to the patient.

Nephrology

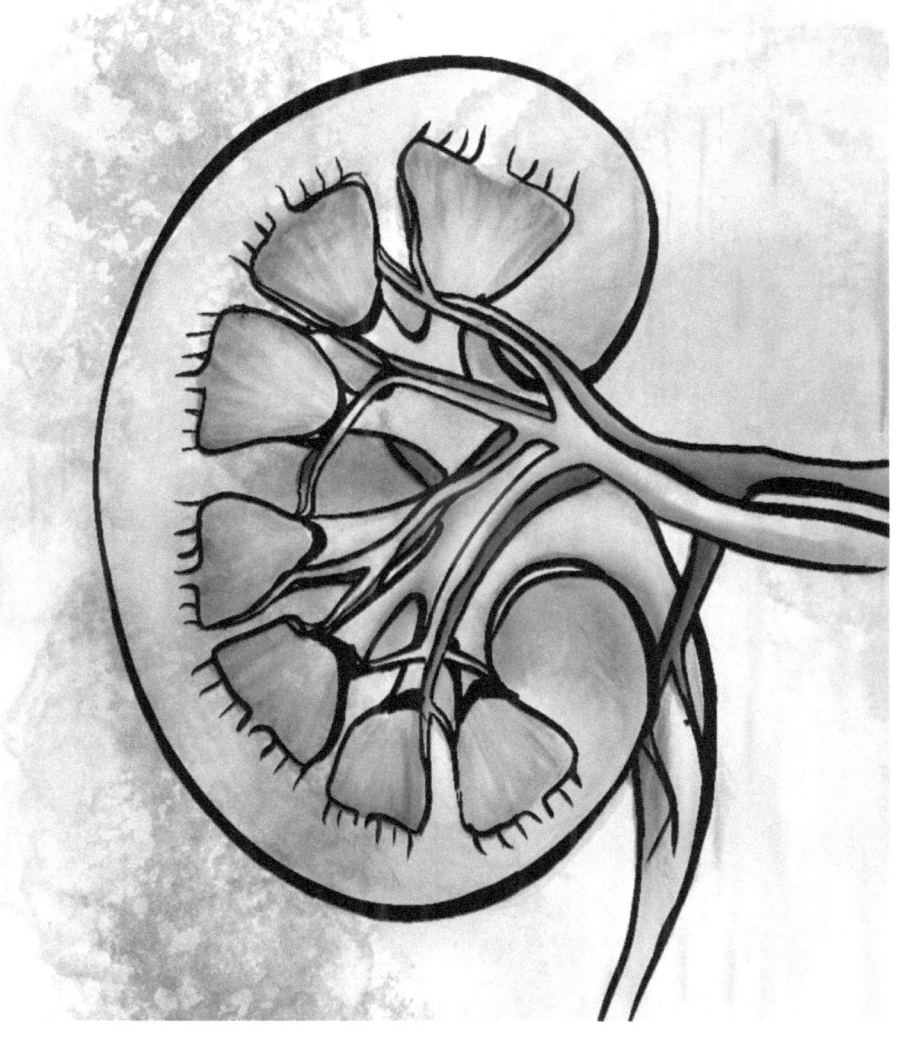

Nephrology
Jinzo-gaku

Constantly adjust
Strong blood flow, pressure a must
For these clean machines

Not a drink yet drunk
Gap, buzz from fermenting funk
Complicated gut
Slurred speech, pH, all befall
Carbs bypass to large from small

D-Lactic Acidosis

D-lactate is the stereoisomer of L-lactate, the form involved in most pathophysiology and regularly measured by laboratory assays. D-lactate is a product of colonic bacterial metabolism and significant D-lactic acidosis can develop in patients with short bowel syndrome, such that ingested carbohydrates are metabolized by colonic flora. Symptoms of D-lactic acidosis include inebriation, stupor, coma, and a high-anion gap acidosis. Diagnosis requires clinical suspicion and measurement of D-lactate, often requiring a send-out to a special laboratory. Treatment includes bicarbonate supplementation, antibiotics, and a low-carbohydrate diet.

Blue plugged into red
Gush of blood detoured instead
Grows ropy and tough
Veins becomes like 'artery'
High flow, buzz thrill, sweet bruit

Arteriovenous Fistula

An arteriovenous fistula (AVF) is constructed for hemodialysis access. A vein is anastomosed to an artery such that arterial flow fills the vein, rapidly returning blood to the right heart. The thin-walled and compliant vein initially dilates but will become thicker-walled and 'arterialized' with continued exposure to increased blood flow. The AV fistula provides arterial flow from the vein for dialysis while reducing the risk of downstream ischemia or embolization into the arterial bed. AV fistulas have a lower infection risk than other forms of hemodialysis access, such as grafts or tunneled catheters, and can provide decades of durable dialysis access.

Life loss Mg and K
Broken channel made that way
Cramping, long QT
Diagnosed late as adult
Constant craving for lost salt

Gitelman Syndrome

Gitelman syndrome, named for Hillel Gitelman (1932-2015), is the autosomal recessive loss or malfunction of the kidneys' thiazide-sensitive sodium chloride (NCC) cotransporter. The syndrome can be symptomatically mild and may be first diagnosed in children or adults. Without the NCC cotransporter, there is volume depletion, hypokalemia, hypomagnesemia, low urine calcium, metabolic alkalosis and chondrocalcinosis. The diagnosis of Gitelman syndrome requires ruling out vomiting and surreptitious diuretic use. Lifelong treatment includes supplementation with sodium, potassium, and magnesium.

Red cells gauntlet run
Shot through fence force of blow gun
Broken skeleton
Bruised and dazed in filtrate space
Mickey ears further debase

Acanthocytes

Acanthocytes or dysmorphic red cells in the urine sediment are one sign of glomerular bleeding. Red blood cells develop 'Mickey Mouse'-like blebs after being pushed through the wall of podocytes and glomerular basement membrane (GBM) which separates the blood and urinary spaces. Dysmorphic red cells are seen in glomerulonephritis, demonstrating the inflammatory disruption of the podocyte/GBM barrier. They can also be seen in thin basement membrane nephropathy.

Eyes puffed overnight
Frothy pee, feet swollen tight
+++ protein
Gloms look pristine under light
EM effaced podocyte

Minimal Change Disease

Minimal change disease is primarily a pediatric glomerulopathy, though both primary and secondary forms are seen in adults. Secondary causes include NSAIDs, lymphoma and Hepatitis C infection. A subset of cases has a pathologic anti-nephrin antibody. The clinical picture of minimal change disease is one of sudden onset nephrotic syndrome with face and leg edema, heavy proteinuria, hypoalbuminemia and lipiduria. The glomerulopathy is rapidly responsive to steroids, though additional immunosuppression may be required to treat relapsed disease. Minimal change disease is named for the normal appearance glomeruli have under light microscopy, while podocyte effacement is evident under electron microscopy.

Words to be wiser
Do not gulp sanitizer
Though intoxicates
Osm gap without AG
Risk shock, GI injury

Isopropyl Alcohol Ingestion

Isopropyl alcohol ingestion is characterized by inebriation and the presence of an osmolal gap without an anion gap. Patients may have a fruity smell as the alcohol is metabolized to acetone. Isopropyl alcohol is one of two alcohols (with ethanol) permitted in hand sanitizers. Through either accidental or intentional ingestion, isopropyl alcohol can cause gastritis, lung injury, shock, and coma. Patients are given supportive management.

High K, low Aldo
Buffering production slowed
Rare ammonia
Protons accrue without trap
pH lowered but no gap

Type 4 Renal Tubular Acidosis

Type 4 renal tubular acidosis (RTA) is a normal anion gap metabolic acidosis with hyperkalemia and/or aldosterone deficiency or resistance. Production of the buffer ammonia (NH_3) is impaired, limiting the excretion of urine ammonium (NH_4^+), a major renal mechanism for clearing acid. There are many etiologies for Type 4 RTA including diabetic renal disease, angiotensin inhibitors, IV heparin, and primary adrenal insufficiency.

World had grown too bleak
Wood spirit drunk, vision weak
Swollen optic disc
Rash search for life more placid
Leaves blind from formic acid

Methanol Poisoning

Methanol ingestion initially causes inebriation and sedation. Its metabolism, through alcohol dehydrogenase, forms toxic formic acid, also known as formate. Formate causes severe retinal injury with optic disc hyperemia, edema, and eventual permanent blindness. It also injures the basal ganglia. An afferent pupillary defect is a sign of advanced methanol poisoning. Poisonings are usually diagnosed clinically, though definitive diagnosis can be made through gas chromatography. While awaiting the lab result, however, patients should receive alcohol dehydrogenase inhibition with fomepizole. Hemodialysis can rapidly remove both the parent alcohol and its toxic formic acid metabolite.

Extra cells in light
EM tubules jammed in tight
Blood and protein spilled
Whirled sheaves, oft from B cell clone
Ruined kidneys' roots are shown

Immunotactoid Glomerulopathy

Immunotactoid glomerulopathy is a rare renal disease characterized by the deposition of organized microtubules into glomerular tissues. It is also called GLOMMID for glomerulonephritis with organized monoclonal microtubular immunoglobulin deposits. Kidney biopsies are Congo Red negative. Patients present with hematuria, nephrotic syndrome, hypertension and reduced glomerular filtration. Light microscopy often shows a membranoproliferative glomerulonephritis picture. Large, orderly microtubules are seen with electron microscopy. The disease may be idiopathic or, more often, due to chronic lymphocytic leukemia, a B-cell lymphoma or multiple myeloma.

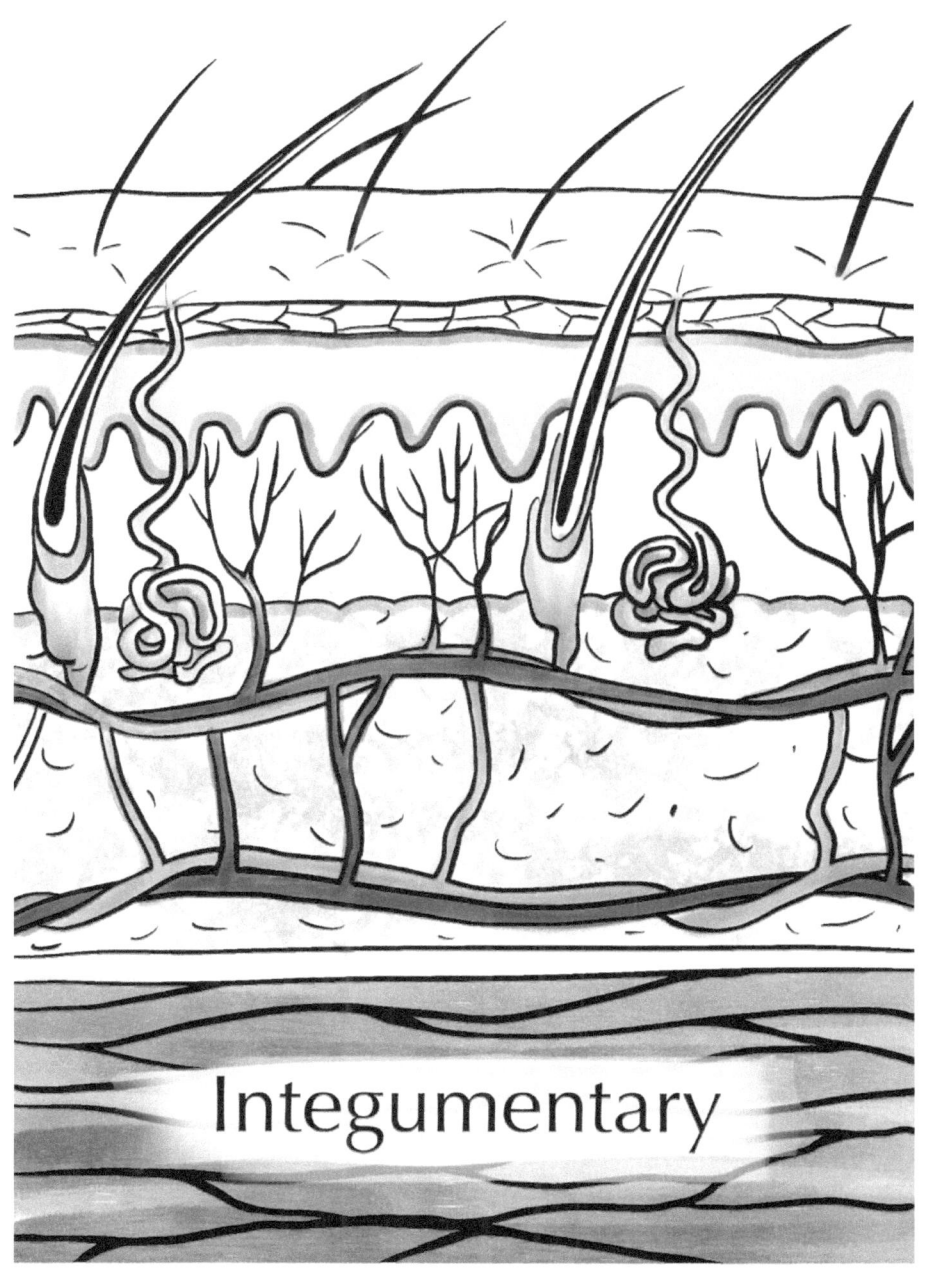

Integumentary
Gaihi

Tall, small, wide, or thin
Structure shapes the size one's in
Vital packaging

Everything's too loud
Whispers shout like roar of crowd
Whoosh my eyeballs roll
Canal (canal) cover missed
Audio control dehisced

Superior Semicircular Canal Dehiscence Syndrome

Superior semicircular canal dehiscence (SSCD) syndrome is rare. It presents with hyperacusis, autophony (hearing one's heartbeat, swallowing, eye movements), echoing, vertigo or syncope from sound, also known as the Tullio phenomenon. The rift in the covering allows pressure into the canals, causing auditory and vestibular symptoms. Surgical repair is indicated.

Morbid circle sign
Peril lurks beneath waistline
Hemorrhage within

Cullen Sign

The Cullen sign, named for the English gynecologist Thomas Stephen Cullen (1869-1953), is described as superficial edema and bruising in the subcutaneous fatty tissue around the umbilicus. The sign was originally described in association with ruptured ectopic pregnancy. It has since been associated with many retroperitoneal pathologies, including acute pancreatitis, splenic rupture and perforated duodenal ulcer. Blood diffuses from the retroperitoneum along the gastrohepatic and falciform ligaments to stain tissues around the umbilicus.

Grooves trauma inscribed
Keratin marks life survived
Arrest, growth beyond

Beau's Lines

Beau's lines are named for Joseph Honore Simon Beau (1806-65), a French physician famed for physiologic studies of the heart and lungs. Beau's lines are transverse nail lines, consistent with a growth arrest. This arrest may reflect a time of illness or a toxic exposure, such as chemotherapy.

Chemo, just a dash
Linear distinctive rash
Dark slash marks each scratch
Strong pruritus can precede
Stop drug, whip rash will recede

Similar linear bloom
Post raw shiitake mushroom

Flagellate Dermatitis

Flagellate dermatitis is a linear, pruritic rash marked by areas of erythema or hyperpigmentation at areas of scratching. The rash has been most often associated with the chemotherapy drug Bleomycin. A similar rash occurs after the ingestion of raw shiitake mushrooms.

Arch's chandelier
Hard palate with ridged veneer
Touch point for the tongue
Blunt stalactite one can see
Mass is fixed unlike PB

Torus Palatini

Torus palatini are hard, benign growths on the roof of the mouth. They are more common in women and in Asian populations. These growths are usually asymptomatic but can interfere with swallowing or the fit of dentures. PB is a shortening of peanut butter, which also sticks to the roof of the mouth, if only temporarily.

Tongue cartography
White red edge marks land and sea
World all in their head

Geographic Tongue

Geographic tongue, also known as benign migratory glossitis, is due to recurrent inflammation of the dorsal tongue. Loss of filiform papillae creates red patches with white, circumferential borders. This pattern gives the tongue the appearance of a map. Lesions are migratory such that the pattern is constantly changing. Patients can have numerous flares and remissions. Most patients are asymptomatic or may have discomfort or sensitivity to acidic or spicy foods.

Heating pad held tight
Constant warmth clutched close each night
Skin brown fishnet square

Erythema Ab Igne

Erythema ab igne is a reticular, hyperpigmented dermatosis which occurs in response to repeated exposure to moderate heat or infrared radiation. These lesions may occur after occupational exposures, e.g., bakers, glassblowers, from prolonged use of heating pads or heated car seats, or from the habit of resting one's computer on the thighs. The lesions may resolve spontaneously with removal of the heat source or become permanently hyperpigmented.

Dribble, plant, quick turn
Foot sticks, leg twists, pop and burn
Hobble hop to side
Top draft pick, no more to score
Pull: loose anterior drawer

Anterior Cruciate Ligament Tear/Ant. Drawer Sign

Anterior cruciate ligament (ACL) tear is evidenced by a positive anterior drawer sign. The typical mechanism for this injury involves a jumping or running athlete who suddenly stops and changes direction. The pivoting motion results in pulling the tibia forward on the femur. Sports associated with ACL injuries include soccer, basketball, skiing, and tennis. The tear may also occur after a direct blow which hyperextends the knee. Patients often note a 'pop' in their knee at the moment of injury, followed by swelling and a sense of instability. The anterior drawer test is one sensitive bedside test for detecting an ACL tear.

Trauma leaves its mark
Behind the ear, plum and dark
Hidden rift skull base

Battle Sign

Retroauricular bruising, the 'Battle sign', named for William Henry Battle (1855-1936), and periorbital ecchymoses, the 'raccoon eyes sign', are superficial signs of a skull base fracture. Fractures may involve any of the five bones that comprise the skull base, but most often involve the temporal bone. Fractures may cause a dural tear and subsequent cerebral spinal fluid (CSF) leaks, presenting as CSF rhinorrhea or otorrhea. Urgent neurosurgical consultation, often with otorhinolaryngology and oromaxillofacial surgery, is indicated.

Lumpy, reddened schnoz
Chronic fire of unknown cause
Deforms central face

Rhinophyma

Rhinophyma is a complication of the skin condition rosacea. The 'phymatous' changes of rosacea include tissue hypertrophy, dilated follicles, and irregular nodular growths. The nose is affected most often, but the cheeks, chin and ears may also be involved. Treatment often includes months of topical isotretinoin. Laser ablation or cosmetic surgery may be necessary to remove the growths and/or recontour the features.

Lost slide, rough rhythm
Stuck tendon pulley system
Snap! Finger triggered
Sharp palm prick and steroids spread
Grease 'wheels', digit works again

Trigger Finger

Stenosing flexor tenosynovitis, also known as a 'trigger finger,' localizes to the retinacular pulley system overlying the metacarpophalangeal (MCP) joint. The flexor tendon catches as it slides through a stenotic sheath, resulting in a loss of the glide to flexion and extension of the finger. The finger may become locked in flexion or extension and require manipulation to unlock. Trigger finger can be a sign of underlying diabetes mellitus or hypothyroidism. Local glucocorticoid injections may help to restore normal sliding. Surgical release is rarely necessary for triggering that persists despite injections.

Small rock thrown at face
Red pool's slow rise fills eye space
Dark horizon climbs

Hyphema

Traumatic hyphema, or visible blood in the anterior chamber of the eye, is often a complication of blunt or penetrating injury. The mechanism of injury may be low energy, such as being hit by a ball during sport, or high-energy, as in paintball injuries or airbag deployment. Spontaneous hyphemas can occur in diabetes mellitus, sickle cell anemia, clotting disorder such as hemophilia, or with the use of antiplatelet or anticoagulant medications. Patients with hyphema should have an ophthalmologic evaluation.

Polygonal lumps
Purple, itchy, flat-topped bumps
Wickham's striae top

Lichen Planus

Lichen planus involves skin and mucous membranes with an eruption of flat-topped, violaceous plaques and papules. The 5Ps mnemonic for lichen planus is pruritic, purple, polygonal, plaques and papules. Lichen planus has a close association with hepatitis C infection but can also be seen in chronic non-HCV-related hepatitis and primary biliary cirrhosis. The lichen planus lesions have characteristic fine whitish lines across their tops, called Wickham's striae, named for Louis Frederic Wickham (1861-1913).

Arcing across eye
Webbed response to too much sky
Wispy winging blinds

Pterygium

Pterygium, Greek for 'wing', is also called 'Surfer's Eye.' Vascular tissue grows from corner toward the cornea in response to solar and wind stress. These may be asymptomatic, irritating or blinding if they extend to the cornea. Treatments range from sun protection and lubricating eye drops to surgical resection.

Pop! Odd bulge to arm
Too much lifting caused this harm
So much for spinach
Could be tendon pulled too far
Or first sign ATTR

Popeye Sign

The 'Popeye Sign' denotes biceps tendon rupture, with bunching of the muscle mid-upper arm with flexion. This rupture has been associated with senile cardiac amyloidosis and the deposition of a protein derived from transthyretin (TTR).

Burnt, black blisters burst
Trunk, limbs, lips, lids, eyes the worst
Start of AED
Case mistaken identity
Rapid stop of drug is key

SJS/TEN

Stevens Johnson Syndrome/Toxic Epidermal Necrolysis are severe drug reactions distinguished by the percentage of body surface area (%BSA) involved. These blistering reactions involve skin and mucosal surfaces. The drugs most often implicated are the anti-epileptic drugs (AED), sulfa antibiotics, allopurinol and NSAIDs. Treatment involves discontinuation of the drug and specialized burn management.

Strong bisphosphonate
Coats bones, shields from morbid fate
Exposed mandible
Gums neglected, molars loose
Do extractions before use

Osteonecrosis of the Jaw

Medication-Related Osteonecrosis of the Jaw (MRONJ) is a serious side effect from the use of osteoclast inhibitors, such as high-potency bisphosphates and denosumab, as part of cancer treatment. Areas of exposed and necrotic bone are the characteristic lesion of MRONJ. Symptoms include jaw pain, gingival inflammation, and fistulae. Treatment is usually conservative with antibiotic rinses and limited intervention. Prevention includes dental evaluation before, with extractions if needed, the start of osteoclast inhibitor treatment and subsequent close dental follow-up during their use.

Failure to protect
Skin mutations now project
Spines of keratin
Solar stress alters skin genes
Talons sprout like wolverines'

Cutaneous Horns

Cutaneous horns (*Cornu cutanerum*) are growths of keratin, often from a base of actinic keratosis but may arise from squamous cell carcinomas. These resemble animal horns, having more height than their base radius. The horns are often small but can grow massive in size. Cutaneous horns are likely due to accrued solar damage and occur most often in elderly patients.

Startling blood splash
Dry heave, hard cough, red-white clash
Eyeball horror show
Painless, glistening, garnet lake
No trauma? Few steps to take

Subconjunctival Hemorrhage

A subconjunctival hemorrhage is a clear demarcated area of extravasated blood under the thin, transparent conjunctiva. This may occur spontaneously or due to a Valsalva maneuver associated with coughing, sneezing, or vomiting. Patients have no change in vision and are asymptomatic. The blood resorbs over one to two weeks. Recurrent subconjunctival hemorrhage can be seen with anticoagulant therapy, and can suggest an underlying bleeding disorder, if otherwise unexplained.

Rash topography
Charts a bleak biography
Sinister spirals

Erythema Gyratum Repens

Erythema gyratum repens is a rare paraneoplastic rash usually associated with breast, lung, or esophageal cancer. The rash is dramatic and geometric, appearing as polycyclic erythematous plaques that are often pruritic. The appearance is similar to a topographic map. Symptomatic treatment includes topical steroids and anti-pruritus medications, such as gabapentin. Cure of the underlying cancer results in resolution of the rash.

Collagen Type I
Defect, structure comes undone
Sham integrity
Bones, teeth, tendons lose their glue
Early sign sclera shade blue

Osteogenesis Imperfecta

Osteogenesis imperfecta (OI), meaning 'imperfect bone generation,' is a group of genetic disorders with mutations involving Type 1 collagen, resulting in either a deficiency of collagen or poor collagen formation. The main symptom of OI is fragile, low mineral density bones which frequently fracture. Lack of collagen in the sclera of the eye accounts for their 'blue' coloring. Patients often have systemic symptoms, such as hearing loss, cardiovascular complications, pulmonary insufficiency, and constipation.

Splash of pale paint spots
Immune destruction in blots
Lost pigment of skin
Marker autoimmune state
Thyroid, beta cells, bald pate

Vitiligo

Vitiligo is an acquired loss of pigmentation which leaves patches of skin devoid of melanocytes, most evident in patients with dark skin color. It is associated with many autoimmune diseases, such as Hashimoto's thyroiditis, Type I diabetes mellitus and alopecia areata, suggesting vitiligo also has an autoimmune etiology. Repeated mechanical trauma can trigger vitiligo patches, the 'Koebner phenomenon', with this reaction most often seen on the neck, elbows, and ankles.

Do South Pole penguins
In their constant Summer sun
sport yellow eye spots?

Pinguecula

A pinguecula is an accumulation of fat and protein under the conjunctiva, appearing as a yellowish lesion at the limbal conjunctiva. Like pterygium, pinguecula form in response to sun, wind and/or dust exposure. Unlike a pterygium, a pinguecula remains confined to the conjunctiva with no extension to the cornea.

Fever flushes skin
Neutrophils boil up within
Painful eruptions
Vessels spared from these attacks
Angry plum nodular plaques

Sweet Syndrome

Sweet syndrome, first described by Robert Douglas Sweet (1917-2001), is an acute febrile neutrophilic dermatosis marked by painful violaceous nodules and plaques, usually found on the neck or upper extremities. Biopsy of the plaques shows no evidence of leukocytoclastic vasculitis. With the syndrome, there may also be arthralgias and oral ulcerations. Sweet syndrome can be idiopathic or triggered by infection, inflammatory bowel disease, pregnancy, or malignancies, such as acute myelogenous leukemia. Resolution is rapid with steroid treatment.

Gynecology & Genitourinary

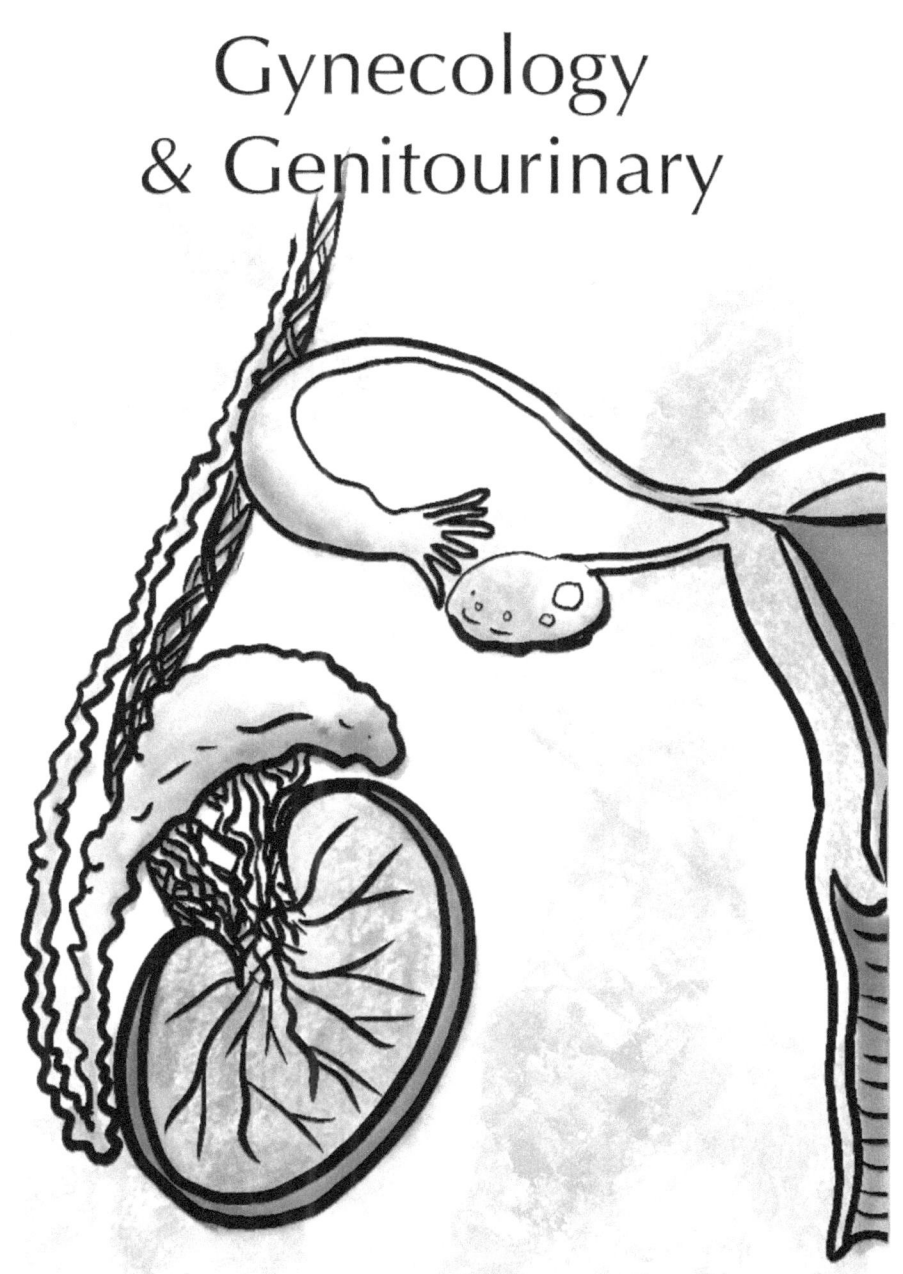

Genitourinary/Gynecology
Hinyoseishokuki/Fujin-ka

Central sites of sex
Complimentary, complex
Excrete, grow anew

Perhaps bladder mass
Blocked and kinked, urine can't pass
Or just huge prostate
Ureters like long balloons
Cortex lost if not popped soon

Bilateral Hydronephrosis

Bilatera hydronephrosis comes from the blockage of both ureters, often by the same process. Kidney stones are a common cause of intra-ureteral obstruction. Causes of extra-ureteral obstruction include retroperitoneal fibrosis and extrinsic tumors. The bladder may be a unifying site of obstruction due to a mass or inflammatory process involving both ureteral openings. Finally, urethral pathology may lead to obstruction of the entire urinary system, either from an enlarged prostate in a man or strictures in either a man or woman. Rapid release of the obstruction is necessary to avoid permanent kidney damage.

GYN nightmare
Goo-filled mass with teeth and hair
Monster barely leashed
Most grow silent, subtle weights
Twist, spill, creature animates

Teratoma

Teratoma is a word coined by Rudolf Virchow (1821-1902), derived from the Greek *'teras'*, meaning monster. Teratomas are tumors composed of multiple cell types derived from all three germ layers. Mature teratomas are the most common ovarian tumor in females in their second and third decades of life. Rarely, these tumors may undergo malignant transformation and, when discovered, should be completely resected.

Days around menses
Knife beneath breast, breath's unease
Dark brown dots thorax
Pleura's chest wall hold unclasped
Scrape, suppress cyclic collapse

Catamenial Pneumothorax

Catamenial pneumothorax is due to pleural involvement with endometriosis. Endometriosis is a disease of uncertain pathogenesis, potentially due to retrograde menstruation. Endometrial glands and stroma are found outside the uterus, including in the thorax. Patients with catamenial pneumothorax present with lung collapse within days of the start of their menstrual period. Pneumothorax is recurrent due to endometrial glands interrupting the seal between the lung and the chest wall. This activity can be suppressed with oral contraceptive pills, danazol, or aromatase inhibitors but definitive therapy includes surgical scraping of the pleura and pleurodesis.

Sudden painful twist
Catches breath as punched by fist
Wave of nausea
Mute cremaster stroked lightly
Urgent call Urology

Testicular Torsion

Testicular torsion occurs when a testicle twists on its vascular pedicle. The patient presents with sudden severe testicular pain, sometimes with nausea and vomiting. Scrotal exam shows a 'high-riding' asymmetric testicle and an absent cremaster reflex. On Doppler ultrasound, there is absent flow in the affected testicle. Torsion is a surgical emergency with the typical window for salvage being around 6 hours from the onset of pain. About 20-40% of testicular torsion cases end in orchiectomy, with the salvage rate dropping quickly with any delay in surgical intervention.

Not for lack desire
Lovin' feeling, light my fire
Serious soft rock
Blown fuse, blocked pipe, scanty flow
Evening rescued by NO

Erectile Dysfunction

Erectile dysfunction is defined as an inability to acquire or sustain an erection of sufficient rigidity and duration for sexual intercourse. It is a form of male sexual dysfunction which is more common with increasing age. Risk factors include cardiovascular disease, obstructive sleep apnea, diabetes mellitus, obesity, smoking, hypogonadism, depression, and some medications, such as antidepressants, alcohol, and anti-androgen therapy. Phosphodiesterase-5 inhibitors are often initial therapy. The action of these drugs is to increase and accentuate nitric oxide-induced penile blood flow by delaying the catabolism of cyclic-guanosine monophosphate (c-GMP).

Cell clump lodged wrong place
Divide, stretch too small a space
Rupture, rent and bleed
Sudden sharp low quadrant pain
Blood lost as torrential rain

Ectopic Pregnancy

Ectopic pregnancy is an extrauterine pregnancy, most often occurring in the fallopian tube, but can be found throughout the abdomen. The most common presentation is first trimester vaginal bleeding and abdominal pain, typically six to eight weeks after the last normal menstrual period. The pregnancy is diagnosed by elevated beta—human chorionic gonadotropin (b-hCG) levels but ultrasound findings of an empty uterus. The feared complication of ectopic pregnancy is rupture of the fallopian tube. This rupture usually presents with severe abdominal pain and signs of a life-threatening intraabdominal hemorrhage.

Ovarian mass
Belly bloats as if by gas
Stage 4 tumor scare
Fluid stretched to pleural space
Fibroma plucked, all erased

Meigs' Syndrome

Meigs' syndrome, named for gynecologist Joe Vincent Meigs (1892-1963), is rare. The syndrome is a triad of ascites and pleural effusion associated with a benign ovarian fibroma. When the fibroma is resected, the fluid resolves. The mechanism for Meigs' syndrome is unclear with one theory of altered capillary permeability due to fibroma's hormone production. Pseudo-Meigs consists of a similar clinical picture with other tumors, including mature ovarian teratoma, struma ovarii, ovarian leiomyomas, and malignant masses.

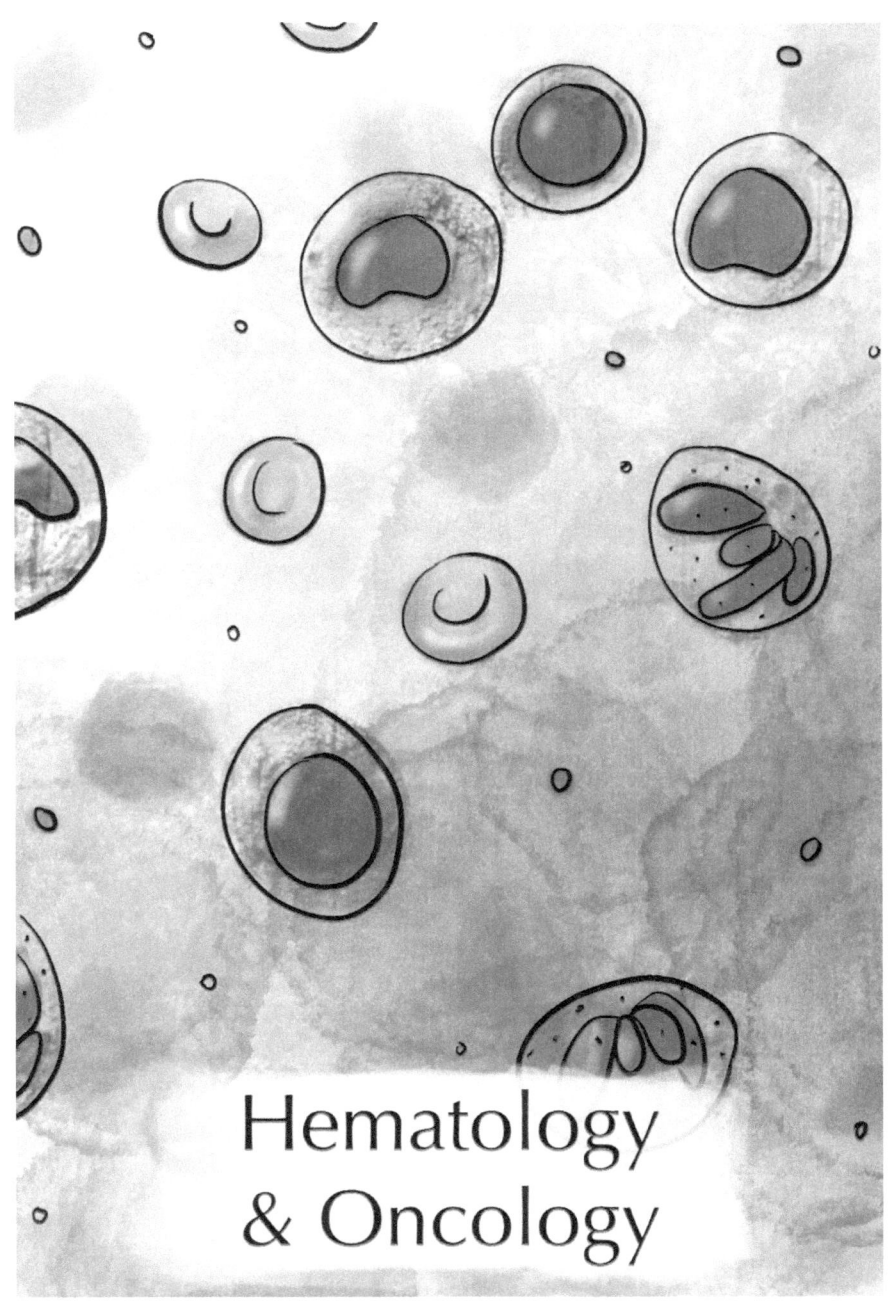

Hematology & Oncology

Hematology/Oncology
Ketsueki-gaku/Shuyo-gaku

Fast-dividing cells
Benign, malign, parallels
Oft shared specialty

In midst of attack
Hepcidin holds iron back
Price of war effort
Red cells right size, numbers lack
Quell the fire, marrow snaps back

Anemia of Inflammation/Chronic Disease

Anemia of inflammation or chronic disease is a common cause of low red blood cell (RBC) counts. Inflammation leads to increased hepcidin activity which subsequently limits both iron absorption from the gut and iron liberation from macrophages. The result is low red blood cell production. The typical RBC profile is a normocytic anemia with a low reticulocyte count and a high ferritin. Treatment of this anemia focuses on resolving the underlying inflammatory disorder.

Young man's nagging hack
Wide white circles float in black
Ugly chest X-ray
Lungs packed cannon balls shot through
Ordnance launched North from GU

Cannonball Metastases

Cannonball metastases are large, well-defined spherical nodules scattered over both lungs. The malignant differential for this pattern of spread includes choriocarcinoma, renal cell carcinoma, prostate cancer, and endometrial cancer. Non-malignant causes of similar shape include *Mycobacteria tuberculosis*, sarcoid and granulomatous polyangiitis. The 'young man' thread in the poem points to 'GU' or genitourinary source for the cannonballs, namely a choriocarcinoma, a rare aggressive form of testicular cancer.

Startling white count
Special slide, smear blood, glass mount
Delicate blue smudge
Few nodes, small spleen, lines preserved
Feeling well, close watch, observe

Chronic Lymphocytic Leukemia

Chronic lymphocytic leukemia (CLL) is characterized by a high count of small blue lymphocytes with tortoise shell chromatin. Cells are fragile and easily disrupted during blood smear preparation, leaving smudge or basket cells on the slide. CLL is common, representing about 25% of all adult leukemias in the United States. Patients are typically older and may be asymptomatic or present with B symptoms (fever, chills, night sweats, weight loss), lymphadenopathy, splenomegaly, or hyperviscosity. Patients without symptoms and a low-risk profile are often just observed.

Hairy nephrosis
Painful long bone sclerosis
Odd histiocytes
Infiltrate, encase, squish, spread
Mutant *BRAF* a common thread

Erdheim Chester Disease

Erdheim Chester disease (ECD) was named for Jakob Erdheim (1874-1937) and William Chester. This rare disease involves clonal non-Langerhans histiocytes which widely infiltrate tissues including bone, kidney, pituitary, and lung. Clinical features can include central diabetes insipidus, bone pain from long bones, eye pain with redness and bulging, weight loss, fever, and chills. Imaging of bones show sclerotic lesions. On cross-sectional imaging, the kidneys appear hairy due to perirenal infiltration and thickening of the fibrous tissue between the renal capsule and perirenal fascia. Many patients have a *BRAF* mutation and may have improvement of disease with targeted treatment.

Packed strands give a sheen
Birefringent, apple green
Proteinaceous path
Stiff, brittle, bruises splatter
Swollen tongue, invasive matter

Red cells line up in rouleaux
Thickened heart but voltage low

AL Amyloidosis

AL amyloidosis is due to deposition of light (and occasionally heavy) chain fragments, derived from a plasma cell dyscrasia, into the tissues of the body. Patients present with widespread organ involvement including renal, nerve, gastrointestinal, tongue and heart. The infiltration expands these tissues and leads to dysfunction such as proteinuria, neuropathy, tongue enlargement and heart failure. Additional clinical features which suggest amyloid are rouleaux formation on blood smears and an infiltrative cardiomyopathy pattern of thickened heart chambers on echocardiogram, but low voltage on ECG. Diagnosis is made by measurement and electrophoresis of serum proteins and by tissue biopsy, demonstrating 'apple green' amorphous deposition with Congo Red stain.

Toes and nose, blanched skin
Purple splotches dot each shin
Frostbite nips at tips
B cell clone's cruel means of harm
Send the test, keep sample warm

Type I Cryoglobulinemia

Type I cryoglobulinemia is most often due to a monoclonal immunoglobulin from a monoclonal gammopathy of clinical significance (MGCS) or a B-cell malignancy such as multiple myeloma, Waldenstrom's macroglobulinemia or chronic lymphocytic leukemia. The immunoglobulins undergo reversible precipitation at low temperature such that the acral parts of the body, e.g., nose, ears, fingers, toes, are most affected. Symptoms result from hyperviscosity, vascular occlusion and gangrene. Therapy is directed at the underlying lymphoproliferative disorder.

Eating in a fret
Paint, ice, dirt, or cigarette
Low hematocrit
Cravings turned to deviancy
From a shortage of Fe

Pica

Pica is named for the magpie (*Pica pica*), a bird known for unusual and indiscriminate eating habits. Pica refers to the eating of non-nutritive substances. Subtypes of pica include pagophagia (ice), clay (geophagia), starch (amylophagia), lead paint chips (plumbophagia) and cigarette butts. Pica is often associated with iron-deficiency and may be exacerbated by pregnancy. It can also be seen in patients with intellectual disabilities, psychiatric disease, and autism.

SICK, smear schistos spread
Coags black, platelets in red
PLASMIC above 5
ADAMTS13 crux
Don't wait! Steroids, PLEX, ritux

Thrombotic Thrombocytopenic Purpura

Thrombotic thrombocytopenic purpura (TTP) is a thrombotic microangiopathy (TMA) due to severely reduced activity of von Willebrand factor-cleaving protease, ADAMTS13. TTP is characterized by platelet-rich thrombi, microangiopathic hemolytic anemia and end organ damage. Most patients present with non-specific symptoms such as fatigue, dyspnea and petechiae. Mortality is high if appropriate management is not initiated rapidly. The PLASMIC score was designed to stratify patients into low-, mid- and high-likelihood of TTP. Plasma-exchange (PLEX) should be started for probable TTP patients prior to the result of the ADAMTS13 test. Rituximab is often added to provide a durable response.

Spiders splashed on chest
High red cell count, EPO test
Monoclonal spike
Kidneys encased back to front
Intrapulmonary shunt

TEMPI Syndrome

TEMPI syndrome, an acronym for telangiectasias, erythrocytosis/elevated erythropoietin, monoclonal gammopathy, perinephric fluid collections, and intrapulmonary shunts, is very rare with only a few cases reported in the literature. The syndrome completely resolves following plasma-cell directed therapy. supporting the hypothesis that the monoclonal gammopathy is both causal and pathogenic.

Opaque red sphere sea
Osmotic fragility
Black pigment gallstones
Increased lysis with each stress
Parvovirus: pale distress

Hereditary Spherocytosis

Hereditary spherocytosis (HS) is an autosomal dominant defect in red blood cell (RBC) membranes resulting in fragile cells and a Coombs-negative hemolysis. The peripheral smear shows spherocytes. HS is diagnosed using a test of EMA (eosin-5-maleimide) binding, which is reduced in HS, and by the osmotic fragility test. Parvovirus B19 infection of a patient with HS can lead to a transient aplastic crisis with severe anemia. Repeated episodes of hemolysis in HS lead to the formation of bilirubin-laden gallstones, otherwise known as pigment stones.

Back's sudden splatter
Dark, rough-hewn stuck-on matter
Marks evil inside
So portends this oft named sign
Most spots though from age, benign

Sign of Leser-Trelat

The sign, named for Edmund Leser (1828-1916) and Ulysse Trelat (1828-1890), describes the sudden, explosive appearance of seborrheic keratosis (SK) lesions as a sign of an underlying malignancy, most often of gastrointestinal origin. Later accounts note that Leser and Trelat described cherry angiomas rather than SKs in their paper though invocations of the Sign persist. Seborrheic keratoses are common skin lesions with age, giving the Sign of Leser-Trelat a tenuous association with malignancy.

Rat poison by way
Competes with Vitamin K
Vermin bleed to death
Drug thins blood, slow, proficient
Save for those C deficient

Warfarin

Warfarin, named for the Wisconsin Alumni Research Fund, first came into large-scale commercial use in 1948 as a rat poison. Warfarin works as a vitamin K antagonist (VKA) blocking vitamin K epoxide reductase, and resulting in decreased activity of clotting factors II, VII, IX and X, as well as proteins C and S. Patients with Protein C deficiency are at risk for developing warfarin-associated skin necrosis. Warfarin's efficacy can fluctuate with patients' intake of vitamin K-containing foods or their use of antibiotics. Direct-acting oral anticoagulants (DOACs) have replaced VKAs for most indications though they continue to be recommended for mechanical heart valves and 'triple positive' antiphospholipid antibody syndrome.

Hard umbilicus
Inflamed, painful but no pus
Firm ball sent for path
Named for nun's pattern decode
Ugly cells creep deep to node

Sister Mary Joseph Node

A Sister Mary Joseph node refers to a palpable nodule bulging from the umbilicus as a sign of metastasis from an abdominal or pelvic malignancy. The proposed mechanism for spread is via the lymphatics which run alongside the umbilical vein. The sign is named for a Catholic nun who was the surgical assistant of Dr. William J. Mayo (1861-1939) at St. Mary's Hospital in Rochester, Minnesota. She was the first to make the association of the nodule and underlying malignancy, and later became the superintendent of the hospital. Dr. Mayo published an article about the phenomenon in 1928.

Cancer's blaze within
Lymph ducts blocked, dimpled by pin
Breast in flames, orange skin

Peau d'orange

Peau d'orange is French for 'orange skin,' describing a thickened, dimpled appearance. Peau d'orange is seen in several disease processes, including Graves' dermopathy, pseudoxanthoma elasticum and chronic infections. The appearance is due to edematous skin and lymphatics, with tethering by skin follicles and sweat glands. Peau d'orange, when accompanied by rapid breast swelling and red, warm, tender skin, is consistent with an underlying inflammatory breast cancer.

Neurology & Psychiatry

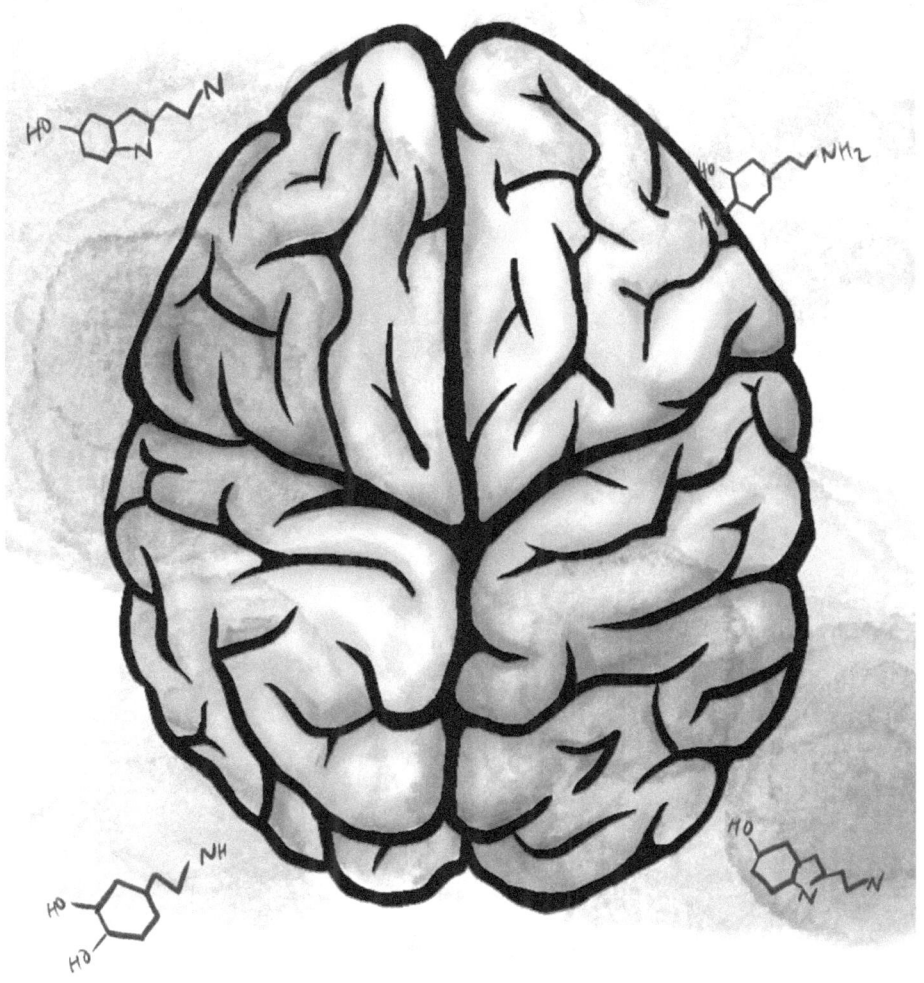

Neurology/Psychiatry
Shinkei seishin igaku

Sum of existence
Total one can think, do, sense
Meta marvelous

Once kind, now pure rage
Vulgar, profane, loosed from cage
Railroad accident
Iron rod through frontal lobe
Blown restraint leaves id disrobed

Phineas Gage

In 1848, Phineas Gage (1823-1860) was a railroad worker when he was involved in an accident which blew a 3'7" tamping iron through his skull. The iron entered under his left orbit and destroyed much of his orbitofrontal cortex. Remarkably, he survived the accident. Reported to be a shy and mild man before the accident, Gage underwent a major personality change and became uncouth, vulgar, and disinhibited. He lived an additional 12 years before dying of seizures. His case sparked many theories about the neuroanatomy and the seat of reason and personality in the brain. Since 1868, his skull and the tamping iron that skewered his brain have resided in the Warren Anatomical Museum at Harvard Medical School.

Blink, blank, mind takes pause
Cortico-thalamic cause
3-Hz spike and wave
Pulsing pushes thoughts aside
First line ethosuximide

Absence Seizure

Absence seizures, also known as generalized non-aware seizures, are more common in children than in adults. The classic seizure is one of repetitive short behavioral arrest, characterized by eyelid fluttering, lip-smacking, or a blank stare, with no post-ictal period. The EEG shows a 3-Hz spike and wave pattern during the seizures. Ethosuximide is the seizure drug of choice.

Sheaf split from within
Fingers numb, pain constant din
Cored out spinal cord
Lore of nymph turned hollow reed
Neurosurgery in need

Syringomyelia

Syringomyelia is a fluid space which develops within the spinal cord. It is associated with Chiari I malformation, tethered cord syndrome, arachnoiditis, scoliosis, and trauma. Patients present with central cord syndrome, which is clinically characterized by loss of temperature and pain sensation with a thoracic syrinx. The syrinx compresses the spinothalamic tract fibers crossing in the central cord. Syrinx may also present with intractable pain. Treatment is surgical fenestration and/or shunt of the fluid collection. The name syringomyelia comes from Greek mythology and the story of Syrinx, the nymph who turned into a hollow reed to escape the lustful attention of the god Pan.

Warped protein in wait
Midlife, sleepless nights stretch late
Dreaming while awake
Hell of night blurs into day
Reaching for sleep, far away

Familial Fatal Insomnia

Familial fatal insomnia is a rare prion disease which demonstrates autosomal dominant inheritance. A few sporadic cases have been reported. The disease is due to a missense mutation of the PRNP gene. The median age of onset is 56 years old, and the disease is rapidly fatal within one year of diagnosis. Symptoms include progressive insomnia, daytime hallucinations, memory loss, spasticity, autonomic dysfunction, and weight loss.

More common less svelte
Squished by belly, band, or belt
Outer upper thigh
Numbness, tingling subacute
Pinprick oval spares the glute

Meralgia Paresthetica

Meralgia paresthetica, Greek for 'thigh pain', is a neuropathy due to entrapment of the lateral femoral cutaneous nerve under the inguinal ligament. Common causes include obesity, pregnancy, ascites, tight belts, and seat belt trauma. The neuropathy is purely sensory with pain and numbness on the upper-outer thigh. The syndrome can be treated with antiseizure analgesics and is usually self-resolving if the compression is relieved. Rarely, patients will require surgical release of the trapped nerve.

Rhythmic twirl of wrist
Hints at cruel genetic twist
CAG repeats
If child's path trails parent's fate
Younger would anticipate

Huntington's Disease

Huntington's disease, named for George Huntington (1850-1916) who first described the disease in detail, is an autosomal dominant progressive neurodegenerative disorder of trinucleotide (CAG) repeats in the Huntingtin (*HTT*) gene. Chorea, psychiatric symptoms, and progressive dementia are clinical features. Imaging shows caudate atrophy. Symptom onset is typically between 30-50 years of age, although subsequent generations may have earlier onset due to 'anticipation' from further expansion of the unstable 'CAG' region of the gene.

Red has lost its zing
Marcus Gunn to flashlight swing
Central scotoma
Painful eye roll, hurts to try
Nerve aflame on MRI

Optic Neuritis

Optic neuritis (ON) is a disease of inflammatory demyelination targeting the optic nerve and optic tract. Most cases are unilateral. Patients present with diminished vision, loss of red color saturation, abnormal pupillary responses to a swinging flashlight test, e.g., a 'Marcus Gunn pupil', central scotoma, and painful eye movements. Funduscopic exam shows blurring of the optic disk margins and hyperemia. Enhancement of the nerve can be seen on contrasted MRI. There is a strong association between ON and multiple sclerosis (MS) and ON may be the first symptom of MS. Ischemic optic neuropathy is a more likely diagnosis in patients >50 years of age and may be arteritic (e.g., Giant Cell Arteritis) or non-arteritic (e.g., ischemia from hypertension or diabetes mellitus).

Fleeting coaster ride
Lips smack, cool stare, blank outside
Dystonic head tilt
Spells conclude with wiping nose
Hippocampus oft sclerosed

Temporal Lobe Epilepsy

Temporal lobe epilepsy is the most common type of focal seizures in adults and is often associated with hippocampal sclerosis. Other causes include tumors, arteriovenous malformations, and perinatal injuries. The seizures often begin with an aura, such as the feeling of being on a rollercoaster, of fear or doom, or a sense of déjà vu. Patients demonstrate automatisms, including lip-smacking or repetitive blinking, which are followed by lateralizing dystonic posturing. The seizure often ends with the ipsilateral hand wiping the nose.

Dazzling light vortex
Released visual cortex
Input lost from eyes
Visions complex in one's mind
'Seen' when sight amiss or blind

Charles Bonnet Syndrome

Charles Bonnet syndrome (CBS), named for the Genevan naturalist (1720-1793), describes visual hallucinations which occur in the setting of low or no vision. The hallucinations are thought to be due to a 'release phenomenon' of the visual cortex from ocular input. CBS is common in patients with age-related macular degeneration, with as many as 1 in 8 reporting symptoms. Patients and their providers may misinterpret hallucinations as a sign of mental illness.

Brain vessels little
Crystallize, stiff and brittle
Crack, split, micro bleed
Anti coag meds may make
Posterior lobar lakes

Cerebral Amyloid Angiopathy

Cerebral amyloid angiopathy (CAA) is characterized by amyloid beta-peptide deposits within small- to medium-sized blood vessels of the brain and leptomeninges. CAA is age-dependent with symptomatic patients nearly all age >60 years old. There is an association with cognitive impairment and dementia. Radiographic findings include microbleeds from and superficial siderosis, or deposition of prior hemorrhagic materials. The most common overt manifestation of CAA is acute lobar intracerebral hemorrhage. The risk of hemorrhage must be considered when weighing the benefits of using antiplatelet or anticoagulation therapy in patients affected by CAA.

Searing burn down arm
Exam free obvious harm
Save winged scapula
From insult a loss of strength
Time to heal nerve mirrors length

Parsonage-Turner Syndrome

Parsonage-Turner syndrome, or neuralgic amyotrophy, is named for the 1948 series by Maurice Parsonage (1915-2008) and John Turner (1911-1980), reporting cases with brachial plexus neuritis involving the long thoracic nerve, with resultant scapular winging. Like Guillain-Barre Syndrome, Parsonage-Turner is often preceded by a viral illness. Patients report intense pain followed by patchy weakness. The acute illness is followed by a slow spontaneous recovery.

Soporific milk
Side effect of Hulk-like ilk
Turns one's urine green

Propofol

Propofol is a short-acting lipophilic intravenous general anesthetic. It is one of several causes of green urine. Others include the drugs methylene blue and amitriptyline. Pseudomonas aeruginosa urinary tract infection can rarely turn urine green.

Pain gnaws deep to eye
Double focus, view awry
Granulomas push
Sided headache, eyeball trapped
Steroids melt tight aching wrap

Tolosa-Hunt Syndrome

Tolosa-Hunt syndrome, named for Eduardo Tolosa (1900-1981) and William Hunt (1921-1999), is idiopathic granulomatous inflammation behind the eye, often involving the superior sulcus and the cavernous sinus. Patients present with unilateral headaches, Pain behind the orbit and cranial nerve palsies, especially ophthalmoplegia. The diagnosis is made by excluding infectious, malignant, and autoimmune causes. There is a rapid response to corticosteroids, but the syndrome may recur.

Slow magnetic gait
Rushing, wet, one cannot wait
Dark spaces dilate
LP drips toward sharper fate
Lost spark, hope shunt sets things straight

Normal Pressure Hydrocephalus

Normal pressure hydrocephalus (NPH) is one cause of reversible dementia. Patients present with a distinctive magnetic gait, bladder incontinence and confusion or dementia. Head imaging shows enlarged ventricles out of proportion to brain atrophy. Lumbar puncture (LP) has a normal opening pressure. In NPH, repeated large volume lumbar puncture results in improvement in gait, and this is part of the diagnostic process. Patients are treated with a surgical ventriculoperitoneal shunt if they show improvement with serial LPs.

Droop to lid on right
Small pupil as in bright light
Same side without sweat
Differential is far flung
Bad path apex of lung

Horner's Syndrome

The poem describes a patient's right-sided Horner's Syndrome, named for Swiss ophthalmologist Johann Friedrich Horner (1831-1886). Horner's syndrome is caused by injury to the sympathetic stellate ganglion with subsequent ipsilateral ptosis, miosis and anhidrosis. The syndrome has a broad differential including trauma, carotid dissection, thyroid disease, multiple sclerosis, and lateral medullary stroke. A feared etiology and classically described cause of the syndrome is a superior sulcus lung cancer invading the ganglion.

Furrowed, stumbling daze
Rigid, fumbling up-down gaze
Midbrain hummingbird
Broad-based gait, oft backward fall
Apathetic, gruff to all

Progressive Supranuclear Palsy

Progressive supranuclear palsy (PSP) is a 'Parkinson's Disease Plus' syndrome characterized by underlying neuropathology involving tau protein deposition and neurofibrillary tangles. It is categorized as a tauopathy. MRI of the brain shows a distinctive 'hummingbird sign' due to atrophy of the superior aspect of the midbrain in the brainstem. Patients present with impaired vertical gaze, bradykinesia, micrographia, a wide-based gait with frequent falls, truncal rigidity and instability, and dementia.

Lose love's worth to you
Illness dements young and cruel
Knife blade atrophy
Pick off clothes, lick a stranger
Gone insight, sense of danger

Frontotemporal Dementia

Frontotemporal dementia (FTD) has an early onset around 50-60 years of age. Patients have prominent behavioral symptoms with apathy or loss of empathy, disinhibition, hyperorality, and compulsive behaviors. MRI imaging shows asymmetric atrophy in the frontal gyri or temporal lobes with a characteristic 'knife blade' configuration of the frontal gyri.

Bloody crescent moon
Burst from bridging veins is hewn
Bruise upon the brain

Subdural Hematoma

Subdural hematoma results from intracranial bleeding between the dura mater and arachnoid membrane, two of the external meninges of the brain. Head trauma is a common etiology, causing tears in venous blood vessels. Risk factors are brain atrophy, infancy, alcohol abuse, and epilepsy. Imaging shows a crescent-shaped accumulation of hyperdense blood. Treatment is based on size of the hematoma and the neurologic examination.

Supernova, pain
Swelling, brain cisterns blood-stained
Hemorrhage within

Subarachnoid Hemorrhage

Subarachnoid hemorrhage (SAH) often causes a 'thunder-clap' headache or the worst headache of life (WHOL) with a sudden onset and severe intensity of pain. SAH is often caused by the rupture of an intracranial berry aneurysm, most commonly on the anterior or posterior communicating arteries of the Circle of Willis. Head CT imaging is notable for an area of bleeding with hyperdense extension to the suprasellar cistern and around the Circle of Willis, the so called 'Star Sign' of SAH.

Flattened nasal crease
Eye stuck open, red, needs grease
Virus? Spirochete?
Brow sags, corneal not brisk
Gravid state at increased risk

Bell's Palsy

Bell's palsy, named for Sir Charles Bell (1774-1842), is a lower motor nerve palsy of cranial nerve (CN) 7. Involvement of the eyebrows and forehead muscles distinguishes it from an upper motor nerve lesion which would only affect the lower half of the face. Potential etiologies for CN 7 palsy include HIV, HSV, VZV, Lyme Disease, sarcoidosis, Guillain Barre Syndrome, Ramsay Hunt syndrome, Melkersson-Rosenthal syndrome, and peri- and post-partum states. When the palsy is idiopathic it is called Bell's palsy. Treatment includes eye care, steroids, and possibly an antiviral depending on the severity. Typical Bell's palsy is self-limited, although rarely it can recur.

Brain's quick twittering
Manic bursts of wit blurring
Cation can quell
Steadiness comes at a cost
Urine's water balance lost

Lithium

Lithium is an alkaline metal, the same chemical category as sodium. It is used as a mood stabilizer and is effective at treating patients with acute mania, hypomania, and bipolar and unipolar depression. Lithium is not metabolized and is primarily excreted in the urine. Systemic side effects of lithium include tremor, thyroid disease, and parathyroid disease. Lithium's similar chemical structure to sodium can lead to renal tubular uptake and toxicity in the forms of nephrogenic diabetes insipidus and progressive renal insufficiency from interstitial nephritis. Patients treated with lithium must have regular laboratory tests to detect renal toxicity and other systemic side effects.

ACKNOWLEDGMENTS

Thank you to the incredibly thoughtful and generous Massachusetts General Hospital resident physicians who helped to refine the poems and assure the explanations were correct: Dr. Hannah Abrams, Dr. Galina Gheihman, and Dr. Dilara Hatipoglu.

Thank you to Sadaharu Honda for the Japanese translation.

Thank you to the wonderful community of #medtwitter for endless inspiration, education and joy in all things Medicine.

Tanka to my tremendous children. Haiku not have done this without you. I love you with all my heart.

INDEX

A
Abdominal aortic aneurysm 32
Absence seizure 314
Acanthocytes 202
Acanthosis nigricans 158
Acute epiglottitis 46
Acute limb ischemia 42
AL amyloidosis 122
Allergic bronchopulmonary aspergillosis 56
Allopurinol 128
Amatoxin-containing mushroom poisoning 174
Amebic meningoencephalitis, primary 74
Anaphylaxis, hymenoptera venom 146
Anemia of chronic disease/inflammation 282
Anterior cruciate ligament tear/ant. drawer sign 230
Anti-synthetase syndrome 120
Aortic coarctation 38
Arrhythmogenic cardiomyopathy 16
Arteriovenous fistula 198
Ascariasis 102
Atrio-ventricular nodal reentry tachycardia (AVNRT) 20

B
B12 deficiency, fish tapeworm 86
Battle's sign 232
Beau's lines 220
Behcet syndrome 130
Bell's palsy 350
Bilateral hydronephrosis 266

C

Candidiasis 108
Cannonball metastases 284
Caput medusae 188
Cardiac myxoma 26
Catamenial pneumothorax 270
Celiac disease 172
Central diabetes insipidus 162
Cerebral amyloid angiopathy 330
Charles Bonnet syndrome 328
Cheyne Stokes respirations 52
Chikungunya 80
Chronic lymphocytic leukemia 286
Ciliary dyskinesia, primary 62
Clostridium perfringens 76
Coccidioidomycosis 70
Courvoisier's sign 180
Cryoglobulinemia, Type 1 292
Cullen sign 218
Cutaneous horns 250
Cryoglobulinemia, mixed 124
Cytomegalovirus 88
Cushing syndrome, paraneoplastic 168
Cutaneous myiasis 92

D

Dermatitis, flagellate 222
Diabetes insipidus, central 162
Dieulefoy lesion 178
Disimpaction, manual 192

Diffuse esophageal spasm 190
Diphyllobothrum latum, B12 deficiency from 86
Disimpaction, manual 192
D-lactic acidosis 196

E
ECG artifact 28
Ectopic pregnancy 276
Epiglottitis, acute 46
Erdheim Chester disease 288
Erectile dysfunction 276
Erythema ab igne 228
Erythema gyratum repens 254
Esophageal spasm, diffuse 190
Esophageal varices 176

F
Fatal familial insomnia 318
Filariasis 104
Flagellate dermatitis 222
Flail chest 60
Frontotemporal dementia 344

G
Gastric antral vascular ectasia (GAVE) 118
Geographic tongue 226
Giardia infection 90
Gitelman syndrome 200

H
Hepatojugular reflex 22
Hereditary spherocytosis 300
Hoover sign 54
Horner's syndrome 340
Huntington's disease 322
Hydatid cyst disease 96
Hydronephrosis, bilateral 266
Hymenoptera venom anaphylaxis 148
Hyperosmolar hyperglycemic state 146
Hyperparathyroidism, primary 156
Hyphema 238

I
Isopropyl alcohol poisoning 206
Immunotactoid glomerulopathy 212

J
Jarisch-Herxheimer reaction 72

K
Kallmann syndrome 152
Kussmaul breathing 48

L
Lactic acidosis, D isomer 196
Legionnaire's disease 82
Leishmaniasis, cutaneous 100
Leprosy 110
Leser-Trelat, Sign of 302
Levamisole 138

Lichen planus 240
Limb ischemia, acute 42
Limited cutaneous systemic sclerosis 136
Lithium 352

M
McConnell's sign 36
Meigs' syndrome 276
Meralgia paresthetica 320
Methanol poisoning 210
Minimal change disease 204
Mirizzi sign 186
Manual disimpaction 192
Molluscum contagiosum 112
Muckle-Wells syndrome 122
Meltzer's triad, mixed cryoglobulinemia 124
Myiasis, cutaneous 92

N
Neurocysticercosis 78
Necrotizing fasciitis, Vibrio 98
Normal pressure hydrocephalus 338

O
Optic neuritis 324
Osteonecrosis of the jaw, medication-induced 248
Osteogenesis imperfecta 256

P
Paget-Schroetter syndrome 44
Paracoccidoidomycosis 84

Paraneoplastic Cushing syndrome 168
Parsonage-Turner syndrome 332
Peau d'orange 308
Pemberton's sign 164
Pericardial effusion 30
Periodic paralysis, thyrotoxic 154
Phineas Gage 312
Phlegmasia cerulea dolens 24
Pica 294
Pinguecula 260
Pityriasis versicolor 114
Pneumothorax, catamenial 270
Pneumothorax, tension 50
Polyarteritis nodosa 140
Polymyalgia rheumatica 134
Popeye's sign 244
Pregnancy, ectopic 278
Primary amebic meningoencephalitis 74
Primary ciliary dyskinesia 62
Progressive supranuclear palsy 342
Propofol 334
Pseudogout 142
Pterygium 242
Pulmonary alveolar proteinosis 58

R
Raynaud's phenomenon 132
Renal tubular acidosis, Type 4 208
Rheumatoid arthritis 126
Rhinophyma 234

S

Scombroid fish poisoning 160
Seizure, absence 314
Sign of Leser-Trelat 302
Sister Mary Joseph node 306
Sporotrichosis 106
Stenosing flexor tenosynovitis 236
Steven Johnson syndrome/Toxic epidermal necrolysis 246
Strongyloides stercolis 68
Subarachnoid hemorrhage 348
Subclavian steal 18
Subconjunctival hemorrhage 252
Subdural hematoma 346
Superior semicircular canal dehiscence syndrome 216
Sweet syndrome 262
Syringomyelia 316
Systemic sclerosis, limited cutaneous 136

T

TEMPI syndrome 298
Temporal lobe epilepsy 326
Tension pneumothorax 50
Teratoma 268
Terminal complement deficiency 66
Testicular torsion 272
Thrombotic thrombocytopenic purpura 296
Thrush 108
Thyrotoxic periodic paralysis 154
Thromboangiitis obliterans 40
Tolosa-Hunt syndrome 336
Torsades de pointes 14

Torus palatini 224
Toxic megacolon 182
Trigger finger 236
Trypanosomiasis 94
Type 1 cryoglobulinemia 292
Twiddler's syndrome 34
Type 4 renal tubular acidosis 208

V
Vibrio vulnificus necrotizing fasciitis 98
Vitiligo 258

W
Warfarin 304
Wolff Chaikoff effect 150
Woltman's sign 166

Z
Zenker's diverticulum 184

www.ingramcontent.com/pod-product-compliance
Lightning Source LLC
Chambersburg PA
CBHW020626220526
45464CB00001B/33